THE Arthritis
HELPBOOK

THE Arthritis
HELPBOOK
What you can do for your arthritis

Kate Lorig, R.N., Dr.P.H.
HEALTH EDUCATOR
STANFORD ARTHRITIS CENTER

James F. Fries, M.D.
ASSOCIATE PROFESSOR OF MEDICINE
STANFORD UNIVERSITY SCHOOL OF MEDICINE

CONTRIBUTING AUTHORS

DEBORAH STINCHFIELD, R.P.T. *Physical Therapist*
INGRID SAUSJORD MOORE, R.D., M.P.H. *Nutritionist*
SHARONA SILVERMAN, M.P.H. *Health Educator*
DORIS MEYER, O.T.R. *Occupational Therapist*
BARBARATERRY KURTZ, M.S.W., M.P.H. *Social Worker*

GRAPHICS SHARON LEIBOLT HATHAWAY

 ADDISON-WESLEY PUBLISHING COMPANY
READING, MASSACHUSETTS ☐ MENLO PARK, CALIFORNIA
LONDON ☐ AMSTERDAM ☐ DON MILLS, ONTARIO ☐ SYDNEY

Library of Congress Cataloging in Publication Data
Lorig, Kate.
    The arthritis helpbook.

    Bibliography: p.
    Includes index.
    I.   Fries, James F., joint author.   II.   Title.
RC933.L63   616.7'22   80-23918
ISBN 0-201-03796-3
ISBN 0-201-03797-1 (pbk.)

ISBN 0-201-03796-3 H
ISBN 0-201-03797-1 P
CDEFGHIJ-DO-89876543210

Third Printing, November 1982

To our 300 group leaders
and to over 4000
Arthritis Self-Management class participants

ACKNOWLEDGMENTS

We would like especially to thank the Stanford Arthritis Center folks: Pat Spitz, Gene Fauro Pratt, Dee Simpson, Beth Kant, Audrey Schomer, R. Guy Kraines, Jim Standish, Alison Harlow, Cathy Williams, Dr. Dennis McShane, Dr. Jeffrey Brown, Dr. Cody Wasner, Dr. Paul Feigenbaum, Dr. Halsted Holman, Dr. Andrei Calin, Dr. Melvin Britton, Dr. Tom Okarma, Dr. William Lages, and Dr. David Schurman. The Midpeninsula Health Service people: Dr. Joseph Hopkins, Judy Staples, Debbie Ridley, Joan Willingham, Jeanne Ewy, Dori Smith, Mary Ann Goodrich, Luann Ciccone, Virginia de Lemos, Sally Semans, and Sarah Reese. The U.C. Berkeley Health Education faculty: Dr. Robert Miller, Dr. Andrew Fisher, Dr. William Griffiths, Dr. Meredith Minkler, Dr. Carol D'Onofrio, and Dr. John Ratcliffe. Significant others: Dr. Robert Swezey, John Staples, Donna Holsted, Carol Rice, Jane Dito, Marie Cascio, Bea Mandel, Dr. Lawrence Green, Dr. Sarah Archer, Janice Pigg, and Carol Simpson. Bonnie Obrig and Sharon Joseph performed yeoman service in manuscript preparation, while Scip Wylbur typed and retyped tirelessly. To all of these fine people our deepest appreciation.

CONTENTS

6

7

8

9

10

11

PREFACE

Before we start we would like to say a little about how this book came to be written and what we have learned in the process.

In 1979 the Stanford Arthritis Center began giving lessons to persons with arthritis. (From the very beginning our class members told us that they did not want to be called "patients.") The classes were taught by 40 people from our community who have arthritis or who are interested in arthritis. With a few exceptions, the teachers were not health professionals. The Arthritis Center staff worked with the teachers, and the lay teachers led the classes.

Our arthritis education classes use the same principles that we have presented earlier in *Take Care of Yourself, Taking Care of Your Child,* and *Arthritis. A Comprehensive Guide,* and they have benefited greatly from the many thousands of encouraging letters and helpful suggestions we have received. In these classes we are not concerned solely with improving knowledge. We also seek to help persons with arthritis change their activities and abilities, decrease their pain, and develop more confidence in themselves as caretakers for their bodies.

In our classes we emphasize three concepts:

1. Each person with arthritis is different. There is no one treatment that is right for everyone.

2. There are a number of things people can do to feel better. These things will not cure most kinds of arthritis, but they will help to relieve pain, maintain or increase mobility, and prevent deformity.

3. With knowledge, each individual is the best judge of which self-management techniques are best for him or her.

Therefore, this book was developed to give details about a variety of self-management treatments. We felt that it was not enough just to know that you should exercise. Instead, you must know about particular exercises, types of exercise, when to exercise, and how much to exercise. You need to understand the relationship between exercise and pain. The same considerations hold for what you need to know about relaxation, nutrition, joint protection, and all other self-management techniques. In *Arthritis. A Comprehensive Guide* we provided all the factual knowledge about arthritis. In this companion volume we try to help you use the information. This is a how-to-do-it book that has been developed with the help of many people very much like you.

When our class members first used this book they liked it but were quick to point out its faults: a neck exercise that caused too much pain, a nutrition section that was unclear, omission of a section on sleep disturbances, and so forth. Taking these suggestions we have added, revised, clarified, re-used, re-revised in a continuing cycle that has resulted in this present edition.

While only seven names appear on the title page as authors and contributors, this book was really written and guided by you, people with arthritis. As of late 1982, more than 4000 people have attended these classes and used this book. From all of them we have gained insights that we hope will be helpful to you.

All these people helped us in other ways, too. We have been carefully studying the effect of our classes on the way that people get along with their arthritis, and our class members have served as the subjects for these studies. In effect we "drew straws" to see which of the subjects on the waiting list would attend the next set of classes and which would have to wait four months. Then we compared how the people who went to the classes did with how the people on the waiting list did. Data from long questionnaires went into the computer, and after elaborate analyses we found what we had suspected all along.

People who exercise regularly (three to seven times a week), practice relaxation, and/or use any of the other self-management techniques have less pain and are more active than those people who are not arthritis self-managers. In addition, these people report that they go to the doctor less often (one and a-half visits less a year). These are the first controlled studies that have ever been done relating education programs in arthritis to outcomes, and they are very encouraging. The bottom line is that arthritis self-managers feel better! We would like to help you become an arthritis self-manager.

Now a few words of caution. First, you did not get stiff, painful joints overnight. Therefore, relief will not come quickly. Self-management is in no way a quick cure; it is a way of life to be practiced every day for the rest of your life. However, it is never too late to start. Our oldest self-manager was 96 when she first came to class.

Second, not everything works for everyone. Experiment, but give each activity two weeks to a month for first results. Don't give up too soon. If one thing does not work for you, try another.

Finally, this book is not meant to replace medical care. Rather, it is a supplement to that care. Most doctors do not have or do not take the time to explain exercises or joint protection in enough detail to help you very much. Therefore, we are hopeful that this book will assist both you and your physician. All of the advice and activities that we describe have been reviewed by many, many doctors, physical therapists, occupational thera-pists, nutritionists, and nurses, including the entire staff of the Stanford Arthritis Center. They represent a sound program essentially the same as that recommended by most health authorities today. If you have particular questions please talk them over with your doctor.

We would like you to feel that you are part of our cast of thousands. If you have comments or suggestions please send them to us by writing:

Stanford Arthritis Center
701 Welch Road, Suite 2208
Palo Alto, California 94304

Your suggestions will be reviewed and considered for our next edition. To all of you who helped in the past and who we couldn't name, many thanks, and to those of you who are just joining, a hearty welcome.

Stanford, California   K. L.

August 1982   J. F. F.

1
Arthritis
WHAT IS IT?

Arthritis. The very word evokes a specter of fear and pain. People think of getting old, being unable to get around, and of becoming more dependent upon others. More so than with any other disease, the term "arthritis" carries with it a sense of hopelessness and futility. But the very opposite should be true. All arthritis can be helped.

In order to understand how to work with your arthritis, it is necessary to know a little about it. In fact, arthritis is not just a single disease. There are over 100 kinds of arthritis, all of which have something to do with one or more joints in the body. Even the word *arthritis* is misleading. The *arth* part comes from the Greek word meaning "joint," while *itis* means "inflammation or infection." Thus the word *arthritis* means "inflammation of the joint." The problem is that in many kinds of arthritis, the joint is not inflamed. A better description might be "problems with the joint."

The next step is to understand what a joint looks like and what the various parts do.

1

WHERE ARTHRITIS ATTACKS

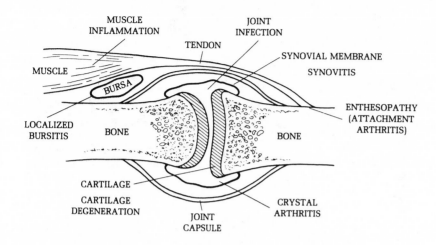

A joint is a meeting of two bones for the purpose of allowing movement. It has the following six parts.

1. **Cartilage.** The end of each bone is covered with cartilage, a tough material that cushions and protects the ends of the bone. To get some idea of what cartilage is like, feel the middle of your nose or your ears. These are also made of cartilage. Cartilage in meat is "gristle."

2. **Synovial membrane (synovial sac).** Around each joint is the synovial sac, which protects the joint and also secretes the synovial fluid, which oils the joint. In fact, this fluid has many times the lubricating power of oil.

3. **Bursa.** A bursa is a small sac that is not part of the joint but is near the joint. It contains a fluid that lubricates the movement of muscles: muscle across muscle and muscle across bones. In some ways it is similar to the synovial sac.

4. **Muscle.** The muscles are elastic tissues that, by becoming shorter and longer, move the bones and thus move you.

5. **Tendon.** The tendons are fibrous cords that attach the muscles to the bones. You can feel them on the back of your hand or in the back of your knee.

6. **Ligament.** The ligaments are much shorter fibrous cords that attach bone to bone and reinforce the joint capsules.

When someone says, "I have arthritis," it means that something is wrong with one or more of these parts. For example, when the synovial membrane becomes inflamed, this is true arthritis. That is, the joint is inflamed. However, if the muscle becomes stretched from overexercise or is injured, this is not arthritis. The joint itself is not affected.

While there are over 100 types of arthritis, we will discuss only two major types—rheumatoid arthritis and osteoarthritis. If you are interested in knowing more about other types of arthritis, read *Arthritis. A Comprehensive Guide*, by Dr. James F. Fries (Reading, Mass.: Addison-Wesley, 1979).

2
Rheumatoid Arthritis
INFLAMED JOINTS

Rheumatoid arthritis (RA) is more than just arthritis. Indeed, many doctors call it "rheumatoid disease" to emphasize its widespread nature. The name is trying awkwardly to say the same thing; the term *rheum* refers to the stiffness, body aching, and fatigue that often accompany rheumatoid arthritis. Persons with RA often describe feeling much like they have a virus, with fatigue and aching in the muscles, except that, unlike a usual viral illness, the condition may persist for months or even years.

About one-half of one percent of our population has rheumatoid arthritis, some one million individuals in the United States. Most of these people (about three-quarters) are women. The condition usually appears in middle life, in the forties or fifties, although it can begin at any age. Rheumatoid arthritis in children is quite different. Rheumatoid arthritis has been medically identified for about 200 years, although bone changes in the skeletons of some Mexican Indian groups suggest that the disease may have been around for thousands of years.

Since RA is so common, and because it can sometimes be severe, it is a major national health problem. It can result in difficulties with employment, problems with daily activities, and can put a severe stress on family relationships. In its most severe forms, and without good treatment, it can result in deformities of the joints. Fortunately, most people with RA do well and lead normal lives. Fear of rheumatoid arthritis, sometimes greatly exaggerated, can be as harmful as the disease itself.

In RA, the synovial membrane lining in the joint becomes inflamed. We don't have a good explanation as to why this inflammation starts, but the cells in the membrane divide and grow, and inflammatory cells come into the joint. Because of the bulk of these inflammatory cells, the joint become swollen, and feels puffy or boggy to the touch. The increased blood flow that is a feature of the inflammation makes the joint warm. The cells release chemicals (called *enzymes*) into the joint space and the enzymes cause further irritation and pain. If the process continues for years, the enzymes may gradually digest the cartilage and bone of the joint, actually eating away parts of the bone.

This then is rheumatoid arthritis, a process in which inflammation of the joint membrane, over many years, can cause damage to the joint itself.

FEATURES

Swelling and pain in one or more joints, lasting at least six weeks, are required for a diagnosis of rheumatoid arthritis. Usually, both sides of the body are affected similarly, and the arthritis is said to be "symmetrical." Often there are slight differences between the two sides, usually the right side being slightly worse in right-handed people and vice versa. Occasionally the condition skips about in an erratic fashion. The wrists and knuckles are almost always involved. The knees and the joints of the ball of the foot are often involved as well, and any joint can be affected. Of the knuckles, those at the base of the fingers are most frequently painful, while the joints at the ends of the fingers are often normal.

Lumps, usually between the size of a pea and a mothball, may form beneath the skin. These *rheumatoid nodules* are most commonly located near the elbow at the place where you rest your arms on the table, but they can pop up anywhere. Each represents an inflammation of a small blood vessel. They come and go during the course of the illness and usually are not a big problem. They do tend to occur in people with the most severe kinds of RA. Rarely, they become sore or infected, particularly if they are located around the ankle. Even more rarely, they form in the lungs or elsewhere in the body.

Laboratory tests sometimes can help a doctor recognize rheumatoid arthritis. The *rheumatoid factor* or *latex fixation* is the most commonly used blood test. Although this test may be negative in the first several months, it is eventually positive in about 80 percent of persons with RA. The rheumatoid factor is actually an antibody to certain body proteins and can sometimes be found in individuals with other diseases. Some doctors think that it is a way the body fights the disease, others think that it may play a role in causing the joint damage.

The *sed rate* is another frequently used blood test. This test is called in full an *erythrocyte sedimentation rate* and the name sometimes is abbreviated ESR. It doesn't help in diagnosis, but it does help tell the severity of the disease. A high sed rate (over 30 or so) suggests that the disease is quite active. The joint fluid is sometimes examined in rheumatoid arthritis in order to look at the inflammatory cells or to make sure that the joint is not infected with bacteria.

X-rays are not very helpful in the initial diagnosis of rheumatoid arthritis. It is unusual for changes to be seen in the bones or cartilage in the first few months of the disease, even when it is most severe. X-rays can help the doctor determine if damage to the bones or cartilage has occurred as the disease progresses. Some doctors like to get baseline X-rays to compare with later X-rays; we prefer to minimize the total number of X-rays.

Most people with RA notice problems in parts of their body other than the joints themselves. Usually, these are general problems such as muscle aches, fatigue, muscle stiffness (particularly in the morning), and even a low fever. Morning stiffness is often considered a hallmark of RA and is sometimes termed the *gel phenomenon*. After a rest period or even after just sitting motionless for a few minutes, the whole body feels stiff and is difficult to move. After a period of loosening up, motion becomes easier and less painful. People often have problems with fluid accumulation, particularly around the ankles. Occasionally, the rheumatoid disease may attack other body tissues, including the whites of the eyes, the nerves, the small arteries, and the lungs. Anemia (low red blood cell count) is quite common, although it is seldom severe enough to need any treatment.

There can be unusual features due to the inflammation of the joint membrane. A *Baker's cyst* can form behind the knees and may feel like a tumor. It is just the synovial sac full of fluid, but it can extend down into the back of the calf and may cause pain.

Rheumatoid arthritis is one of the most complicated and mysterious diseases known. It is a challenge to patient and physician alike. Fortunately, the course of RA can be dramatically changed in most individuals. More so than with any other form of arthritis, if you have RA you need to develop an effective partnership with your doctor, as discussed in Chapter 13.

PROGNOSIS (THE FUTURE OF THE DISEASE)

Rheumatoid arthritis is the condition that most people think of when they hear the word *arthritis*. An image that comes to mind is of a person in a wheelchair, with swollen knees and twisted hands. True, most such people have rheumatoid arthritis. On balance, rheumatoid arthritis is the most destructive kind of arthritis known. Erosion of the bone itself, rupture of tendons, and slippage of the joints can result in crippling. But most people with rheumatoid arthritis do very, very much better than this. In fact, only one in six persons with RA develops any crippling or deformities at all. And it is probable that these could have been prevented by good, early treatment.

The course of persons with RA usually falls into one of three patterns. The first, and best, is that of a brief illness lasting at most a few months and leaving no disability; this course is sometimes called *monocyclic*. The second involves a series of episodes of illness, separated by periods of being entirely well. This is sometimes termed *polycyclic* and usually does not result in very much physical impairment. The third, termed *chronic*, is a more constant disease lasting a number of years, sometimes for life. Probably the majority of persons with rheumatoid arthritis have this chronic form, but even here, serious crippling is unusual. At first it is hard to be sure which pattern the disease will follow, but a chronic course is suggested by the presence of the rheumatoid factor in a blood test and is strongly suggested if the condition has continued to progress for an entire year.

Often it is hard for persons with RA and their relatives to appreciate that even the worst forms of rheumatoid arthritis tend to get better with time. The arthritis usually becomes less aggressive. The inflammation (synovitis) is less active and the fatigue and stiffness decrease. New joints are not likely to become involved after several years of disease. But even though the disease is less violent, any destruction of bones and ligaments that occurred in earlier years will persist. Thus deformities usually will not improve, even though no new damage is occurring. Hence, it is important to treat the disease correctly in the early years so that the joints will work well after the disease activity subsides.

TREATMENT

Treatment programs for rheumatoid arthritis are often complicated and can be very confusing. In this section we give the broad outlines for sound management. But the combination of measures best for you needs to be worked out with your doctor. It has been said that the person who has himself for a doctor has a fool for a patient. In many areas of medicine, and for some kinds of arthritis, this is not true—you can do just as well looking out for yourself. But with rheumatoid arthritis you do need a doctor. Indeed, if your rheumatoid arthritis is at all severe, you may want to be seen, at least occasionally, by a specialist in arthritis, a *rheumatologist*.

First, some common sense. Your rheumatoid arthritis may be with you, on and off, for months or years. The best treatments are those that will help you maintain a life that is as nearly normal as possible. Often the worst treatments are those that offer immediate relief. They may allow joint damage to progress or may cause delayed side effects that ultimately make you feel worse. So, you must develop some patience with the disease and with its management. You have to adjust your thinking to operate in the same slow time scale that the disease uses. You and your doctor will want to be anticipating problems before they occur so that they may be avoided. The adjustment to a long-term illness, with the necessity to plan treatment programs that may take months to get results, is a difficult psychological task. It is easy to understand in principle but hard to put into daily action. This adjustment will be one of your hardest jobs in battling your arthritis.

Synovitis is the underlying problem. The inflammation of the joint membrane releases enzymes that very slowly damage the joint structures. Good treatment reduces this inflammation and stops the damage. Painkillers can increase comfort but do not decrease the arthritis. In fact, pain per se helps to protect the joints by discouraging too much use. So, in RA it is important to treat pain by treating the inflammation that causes the pain. By and large, pain relievers such as codeine, Percodan, Darvon, or Demerol must be avoided. (To learn more, read Chapter 12.)

The proper balance between rest and exercise is hard to understand. Rest reduces the inflammation, and this is good. But rest also lets joints get stiff and muscles get weak. With too much rest, tendons become less strong and bones get softer. Obviously, this is bad. So, moderation is the basic principle. It may help you to know that your body usually gives you the right signals about what to do and what not to do. If it hurts too much, don't do it. If you don't seem to have much problem with an activity, go ahead. As a general rule, if you continue to have exercise-caused pain for more than two hours after exercising, you have done too much.

A particularly painful joint may require a splint to help it rest. Still, you will want to exercise the joint by stretching it gently in different directions to keep it from getting stiff. You will not want to use a splint for too long, or you may want to use it just at night. As the joint gets better you will want to begin using the joint, gently at first but slowly progressing to more and more activity. In general, favor activities that build good muscle tone, not those that build great muscle strength. Walking and swimming are better than furniture moving and weight lifting, since tasks requiring a lot of strength put a lot of stress across the joint. And regular exercises done daily are better than occasional sprees of activity that unduly stress joints not ready for so much exertion.

Common sense and a regular, long-term program are the keys to success. Should you take a nap after lunch? Yes, if you're tired. Should you undertake some particular outing? Go on a trip? You know your regular daily activity level. Common sense will answer most such questions. Full normal activity should be approached gradually with a long-term conditioning program that includes rest when needed and gradual increases in activity during non-resting periods.

Physical therapists and occupational therapists can often help with specific advice and helpful hints. The best therapists will help you develop your own program for home exercise and will teach you the exercises and activities that will help your joints. However, don't expect the therapist to do your program for you. Your rest and exercise program cannot consist solely of formal sessions at a rehabilitation facility. You must take the responsibility to build the habits that will, on a daily basis, protect and strengthen your joints. It is important to start exercise and joint protection before you have problems. These are good preventive measures.

Medications are required by most persons with rheumatoid arthritis and often must be continued for months or years. By and large, the most powerful drugs have the worst side effects. So, good physicians will begin with the simplest and the safest drugs and will use more hazardous drugs only if the simpler measures are not sufficient. Most people will not require the more powerful drugs.

Aspirin is the most valuable single drug, when used correctly. Every person with arthritis should know all about aspirin. Aspirin, used correctly, is a strong anti-inflammatory drug with an acceptable level of side effects. Drugs roughly similar to aspirin are called *nonsteroidal anti-inflammatory drugs* and are frequently used. Examples of such drugs are Motrin, Nalfon, Tolectin, Naprosyn, and Indocin. (For more information, see Chapter 12.)

Antimalarial drugs such as chloroquine or Plaquenil are sometimes used next, if the anti-inflammatory agents have not been enough. Gold injections are often helpful if the previous drugs have not been sufficient and sometimes result in complete disappearance of the arthritis. Penicillamine is a fairly new drug that also can result in dramatic improvement.

Corticosteroids, most frequently prednisone, are strong hormones with dangerous long-term side effects. Their use is controversial in rheumatoid arthritis; some physicians feel that they should almost never be used, and others use them, but only in very small doses. Immunosuppressant drugs, such as Cytoxan, Imuran, or chlorambucil, are powerful, experimental, and hazardous; many physicians think that these drugs are too dangerous to use in rheumatoid arthritis. Steroids and immunosuppressants are sometimes needed for severe complications such as nerve damage or eye damage.

Surgery sometimes can restore the function of a damaged joint. Hip replacement, knee replacement, and synovectomy (removal of the joint membrane) are the most common operations.

3
Osteoarthritis

Osteoarthritis (osteoarthrosis, OA, degenerative joint disease, DJD) is the kind of arthritis that everybody gets. It is a practically universal problem, increasing with age, and one that, because of its relationship to the aging process, is not as responsive to medical treatment as we might like. However, there are many things you can do for yourself to help this disease. Fortunately, osteoarthritis usually is a mild condition. Osteoarthritis is a much less severe form of arthritis than rheumatoid arthritis. In other words, the changes in the skeleton that occur with age are inevitable, but they cause symptoms in a minority of people and severe symptoms in very few.

The tissue involved in osteoarthritis is the cartilage. This is the gristle material that faces the ends of the bones and forms the surface of the joint on both sides. Gristle is tough, somewhat elastic, and very durable. The cartilage or gristle does not have a blood supply, so it gets its oxygen and nutrition from the surrounding joint fluid. In this it is aided by being elastic and by being able to absorb fluid. When we use a joint, the pressure squeezes fluid and waste products out of the cartilage, and when the pressure is relieved, the fluid seeps back, together with oxygen and nutrients. Hence, the health of the cartilage depends on use of the joint. Over many years, the cartilage may become frayed and may even wear away entirely. When this happens, the bone surface on one side of the joint grates against the bone on the other side of the joint, providing a much less elastic joint surface. With time, the opposing bony surfaces may become polished, a process called *eburnation*. As this happens, the joint may again move more smoothly and cause less discomfort. This is one of the reasons it is important to continue to use painful joints.

Osteoarthritis is sometimes called osteoarthrosis. The difference between these two terms has to do with the question of inflammation. *Itis* denotes inflammation, and with osteoarthritis very little inflammation is to be found. Hence, some experts prefer the term osteoarthrosis, which does not imply inflammation. Both words mean the same.

There are three common types of osteoarthritis. The first and mildest causes knobby enlargement of the finger joints. The end joints of the fingers become bony and the hands begin to assume the appearance we associate with old age. The other joints of the fingers may also be involved. This kind of arthritis (or arthrosis) usually causes little difficulty beyond the cosmetic. There may be some stiffness.

The second form of osteoarthritis involves the spine. Bony growths (spurs) appear on the spine in the neck region or in the low back. Usually the bony growths are associated with some narrowing of the space between the vertebrae. This time the disc rather than cartilage is the material that becomes frayed. Changes in the spine begin early in life in almost all of us, but cause symptoms relatively seldom.

The third form of osteoarthritis involves the weight-bearing joints, almost always the hips and knees. These problems can be quite severe. It is possible to have all three kinds of osteoarthritis or any two of them, but often a person will have only one.

Individuals who have had fractures near a joint or have a congenital malformation at a joint seem to develop osteoarthritis in those joints at an earlier age. On the other hand, the usual description of this arthritis as "wear and tear" is not accurate. While excessive wear and tear on the joint can theoretically result in damage, activity helps the joint remain supple and lubricated, and this tends to cancel out the theoretically bad effects.

At any rate, careful studies of people who regularly put a lot of stress on joints (such as individuals who operate pneumatic drills or run long distances on hard paved surfaces) have been unable to show a relationship between these activities and the development of arthritis. Hence, intensive activity does not predispose you to arthritis any more than intensive activity predisposes you to heart disease. In fact, the very opposite may be true.

FEATURES

The bony knobs that form around the end joints of the fingers are called *Heberden's nodes* after the British doctor who first described them. In the middle joints of the fingers, similar knobs can be found. Usually, the bony enlargement occurs slowly over a period of years and is not even noticed. In most cases, all of the fingers are involved more or less equally.

Osteoarthritis of the spine does not cause symptoms unless there is pressure on one of the nerves or irritation of some of the other structures of the back. If someone tells you that you have arthritis in your spine, do not assume that the pain you feel is necessarily related to that arthritis. Most people with X-rays showing arthritis of the spine do not have any problem at all.

Osteoarthritis of the weight-bearing joints, particularly the hip and knee, develops slowly and often involves both sides of the body. Pain in the joint may remain fairly constant or may wax and wane over a period of years. In severe cases walking may be difficult or even impossible. Fluid may accumulate in the affected joint, giving it a swollen appearance, or a knee may wobble a bit when weight is placed on it. Usually, in the knee, the osteoarthritis will affect the inner or the outer half of the joint more than the other; this may result in the leg becoming bowed or splayed and may cause difficulty in walking.

X-rays can be helpful in evaluating osteoarthritis. The two major findings on the X-ray are narrowing of the joint space and the presence of bony spurs. X-rays pass right through cartilage. Hence, in a normal joint the X-ray looks as though the two bones are separated by a space. In reality, the apparent space is filled with cartilage. As the cartilage is frayed, the apparent joint space on the X-ray narrows until the two bones may touch each other. *Osteophytes,* or spurs, are little bone growths that appear alongside the places where the cartilage has degenerated. It is as though the body is trying to react to a cartilage problem by providing more surface area for the joint, so as to distribute the weight more evenly. The bony growth provides a larger joint surface, although the new bone is not covered by cartilage. In addition, X-rays can sometimes show the holes through which the nerves pass and indicate whether these holes are narrowed or not.

In contrast to X-rays, blood tests are not very helpful in diagnosing osteoarthritis. There is not anything wrong with the rest of the body, so all the tests are normal.

PROGNOSIS (THE FUTURE OF THE DISEASE)

Prognosis is good to excellent for all forms of osteoarthritis. When you think of an aging process, you tend to think of a progressive condition that will continue to get worse and worse. That is not necessarily the case. Osteoarthritis may get worse for a while and then become stable for a long time. A joint that has lost its cartilage may not function well at first, but with use the bone may be molded and polished so that a smooth and more functional joint is developed. Even in the worst cases, osteoarthritis progresses slowly. You have lots of time to think about what kinds of treatment are likely to help. If a surgical decision is needed, you can consider for some time whether you want an operation or not. Crippling from osteoarthritis is relatively rare, and most persons with osteoarthritis remain essentially free of symptoms.

TREATMENT

Joints should be exercised through their full range of motion several times a day. If weight-bearing joints are involved, body weight should be kept under control. Obesity accelerates the rate of damage. The most helpful exercises seem to be swimming, walking, and bicycling, which are easy, can be gradually increased, and are smooth rather than jerky. Exercise should be regular. Thus, if you start getting some osteoarthritis, it is not a signal to begin to tone down your life, but rather to develop a sensible regular exercise program to strengthen the bones and ligaments surrounding the affected joints and to preserve mobility in joints that are developing spurs. (For details see Chapter 5.)

Drug therapy is much less important. We use it to control the discomfort to a certain extent. Aspirin in moderate doses (or acetaminophen, such as Tylenol) is frequently helpful. Indomethacin and other anti-inflammatory drugs may be helpful for some people, particularly if the osteoarthritis is in the hip or the knee. We try to avoid codeine and other strong pain relievers because pain is a signal to the body that helps protect a diseased joint; it is important that this signal is received. (For details see Chapter 12.)

Frequently some kinds of devices can assist. A cane may be helpful; less commonly, crutches are needed. Occasionally, special shoes or lifts on one side of the foot may be helpful.

Most physicians believe that osteoarthritis may be prevented by good health habits. If you are active, maintain a lean body weight, exercise your muscles and joints regularly so as to nourish cartilage, and let your common sense tell you when you have done too much and something hurts, your joints should last a lifetime. Like exercise of the heart muscle, exercise of the muscles and joints provides reserve for the occasional strenuous activities we all encounter. Exercise builds strong tissues that last a long time.

Injection of osteoarthritic joints with corticosteroids is occasionally helpful, and sometimes removal of some fluid from a joint may help. Unfortunately, injections usually do not help much since there is not much inflammation to be suppressed. Injections should not be frequently repeated, because the injection itself may damage the cartilage and the bone.

Surgery can be dramatically effective for persons with severe osteo-arthritis of the weight-bearing joints. The total hip replacement operation is the most important operation yet devised for any form of arthritis. Practically all individuals are free of pain after the surgery and many walk normally and carry out normal activities. The total knee replacement is a more recent operation that already gives far better results than the knee surgery available just a few years ago. Surgery is not required on an urgent basis, and you and your doctor will want to decide the point at which the discomfort or the limitation of your walking has become sufficiently great so that the discomfort, the costs, and the small risk associated with the operation are warranted.

4

Those Nagging Pains

BURSITIS AND GETTING OLD

Most of the problems we tend to call arthritis don't even involve the joint and really aren't even diseases. This is good news. Painful local conditions involving only one or two parts of the body are almost always just an irritation or injury of that part. After that part is rested or fixed everything is all right again. There is no crippling, no threat to life, no need for dangerous medications. Remember the basic principle: For a local problem use a local treatment. Very seldom will you want to take a medication by mouth for a pain in, say, an elbow.

There are a lot of names for these conditions—bursitis, low back strain, sciatica, metatarsalgia, Achilles tendinitis, heel-spur syndrome, sprained ankle, cervical neck strain, frozen shoulder, tennis elbow, housemaid's knee, carpal-tunnel syndrome, and others. Many people call all of these bursitis, while doctors have other and fancier names for them. But they all are local conditions and are first approached the same way. At first you don't even need a doctor for them, but if they don't respond after six weeks of self-treatment or seem alarmingly severe, be sure to see the doctor.

BURSITIS

A bursa is a small sac of tissue similar to the synovial tissue that lines the joints. The bursa sac contains a lubricating fluid, and the bursa is designed to ease the movement of muscle across muscle or of muscle across bone. A bursa does not connect to the joint space of the nearby joint but is a separate sac. In the grand scheme of things the bursa is just an annoying little body area, but bursae can be very painful when they become inflamed. Usually, only one or two will be inflamed at a time, but bursitis of over 20 bursae can occur, and the problems can come and go over the years.

"Housemaid's knee" is a popular term for *prepatellar bursitis,* in which the bursa in front and just below the kneecap is inflamed. *Olecranon bursitis* occurs over the point of the elbow, and sometimes a fluid-filled sac is visible at that point. *Subdeltoid bursitis* occurs at the shoulder, or more precisely, on the outer aspect of the upper arm just below the shoulder.

Features

Bursitis is inflammation of a bursa and results in localized pain. Sometimes the pain is on both sides of the body, as with both knees. There is pain when the inflamed area is pressed, and heat and redness are common. If the bursa is located close enough to the skin, swelling can be seen. Many bursae, however, are buried deep between muscles.

Bursitis comes on relatively suddenly, within hours to days. It frequently follows injury to the area, repeated pressure on the area, or overuse. In the shoulders, particularly, it may be associated with inflammation of the tendon and can be part of a "frozen shoulder" problem.

Prognosis

Almost all episodes of bursitis will subside within several days to several weeks, but may recur. If the process causing the bursitis is continued, the bursitis may persist, otherwise it follows a normal healing course over a period of one week to ten days. Some people seem more prone to bursitis than others and have recurrent problems throughout their lives. If the affected part is held rigid, some permanent stiffness may result; otherwise no crippling whatsoever should result from bursitis.

Treatment

If the problem is tolerable, treat it with "tincture of time." Wait for the body to control and heal the process. Avoid the precipitating cause. Use drugs very sparingly; the process is local and systemic drugs like aspirin are not very helpful. Resting the part will speed the healing, and you may want to use a sling or other device to increase the rest. Gentle warmth provided by a heating pad or warm bath frequently makes the bursitis feel better. The affected area should be worked through its full range of motion two to four times a day, even if it is a bit tender, to prevent stiffness from developing. Additional techniques described in Chapter 8 may also be helpful. But remember, patience and avoidance of reinjury are the major tactics.

If the discomfort persists for a number of weeks despite the measures outlined above, see the doctor. Often, the doctor will recommend that you continue the same general measures discussed here. Alternatively, an anti-inflammatory drug may be prescribed; these help few people and are generally just a way of buying a little more patience from the patient. Finally, the doctor may inject the bursa with corticosteroids (see Chapter 12). These injections are usually successful and not overly painful. They are relatively free of side effects and most physicians feel that they are appropriate treatment for a local condition that is severe and persistent.

GETTING OLD

Local injuries, like bursitis, are often dismissed as "just getting old, I guess." It is true that more older people than younger people have these problems, and they do have something to do with the way that our bodies age.

But they do not need to happen. These problems are sometimes due to abuse of a body part, as in prepatellar bursitis from scrubbing floors on your knees. Much more frequently, however, they are due to disuse. In our society, as you get older you are expected to be less active. And then you get the kinds of health problems that happen to inactive people of all ages. The relationship between local problems and age is mostly accidental; it is really an association of local problems with inactivity.

So you need to be active. If your muscles are trim and in good tone, your heart and lungs are conditioned, your body weight is normal and constant at that level, and you have a regular exercise program you will have far fewer of these problems, and your body will not grow old as rapidly. These measures will keep calcium in your bones, your bursae free and well lubricated, your tendons firm and strong, and your joint cartilage well nourished.

You can control a lot of the aging of your body. The worst mistake that you can make is to consider bursitis or another local problem to be a signal to slow down. It is a signal to speed up, because your body is drifting out of condition. In the next chapter we go through some of the exercises that will help.

5

Use It or Lose It
EXERCISES FOR YOUR ARTHRITIS

One of the most important things you can do to help your arthritis is to exercise, if you do it right. Unfortunately, many people with arthritis think exercise is harmful. Others become discouraged because progress is slow or their exercises are painful. Maintaining a proper balance between rest and exercise and exercising properly are the keys to a successful arthritis exercise program. Let us examine the benefits of exercise, some basic principles, and the different types of exercise. With this knowledge you can plan a successful and enjoyable program.

BENEFITS OF EXERCISE

There are numerous benefits of exercise, touching many aspects of our physical and psychological lives. It is well known that exercise leads to increased strength and flexibility in the muscles and ligaments surrounding the joints. In addition, research has shown that exercise helps to maintain or increase the strength of bone. More dynamic forms of exercise, such as swimming or walking, have important effects on the heart that promote increased endurance and circulation and fight deterioration of the arteries.

Every tissue in the body requires certain foods or nutrients to work effectively. Most tissues have arteries that bring essential foods to them, but this is not true of the joint cartilage. It is only through movement that nourishment is brought by the synovial fluid to the joint cartilage and that waste products are removed. Thus, exercise promotes good joint nutrition.

An appropriate exercise program can lead to a general sense of well-being and accomplishment. It is easy to feel good about yourself when you are accomplishing the goals of a realistic exercise program. Further, the social interactions encouraged by many forms of exercise are also rewarding.

Exercise is a way we can prevent the loss of function that may accompany arthritis. There is a saying that applies particularly to persons with arthritis: "Use it or lose it." If you do not use a muscle or joint you will lose strength and mobility, and thus, function. If loss of function has already occurred, it is important to remember that it was not lost in one day. Likewise, it cannot be regained in one day. Slow progress is to be expected, particularly if your arthritis is severe or your joint limitations have existed for a long time. Expect some setbacks in any exercise program but keep at it. Your efforts will be rewarded in many ways.

PRINCIPLES OF EXERCISE

When Should I Exercise?

Exercises should be done daily for the rest of your life. It is the "weekend warrior" who gets into trouble with painful strained muscles and ligaments. The only time a joint should not be exercised is when it is inflamed, or "hot" (swollen, red, tender to the touch). The "hot" joint is one of the special exercise considerations for people with rheumatoid arthritis. However, even those hot joints should be gently moved through the full range of motion twice a day.

Find a specific time and place to exercise and make this a part of your daily routine. You will have to decide on the best time, but consider the following: It is best to exercise when (1) you have the least pain, (2) you have the least stiffness, (3) you are not tired, and (4) your medication is having maximal effect. You probably want one such period early in the day, and one later.

What Can I Do to Prepare for Exercise?

Athletes learn that warming up before exercise means a more productive session and helps prevent injuries. Here are some warm-up suggestions.

1. A nice, slow general stretch: Lying in bed, (a) stretch one arm up and then the other, (b) push arms forward, opening hands wide, (c) pull arms

back and close hands, (d) pull knees up and do a few bicycle turns in the air, (e) stretch legs out straight, (f) roll to the side, swinging legs off the edge of the bed, using momentum to help you sit up. This warm-up is helpful when first getting up in the morning and is very similar to what a cat does as it gets up from a rest.

2. Begin your exercise program with small movements in a pain-free range. These movements can be anything from your chosen exercise done less vigorously to a good shake (like a dog shaking). Before walking or jogging do some gentle stretching of the leg muscles.

3. Massage can be used to relax stiff joints and muscles prior to exercise. However, it is best not to deeply massage a "hot" joint.

4. Apply heat prior to exercise. Heat tends to relax joints and muscles and relieve pain. How you apply the heat is up to you. No way is better than another. You do not need special equipment or mineral waters. All of the following are acceptable ways of applying heat. When using heat always test carefully for temperature (the elbow is a good tester) to avoid burns.

   a) Take a long, hot bath. A hot spring, whirlpool bath, or hot tub is nice, but not necessary. Use caution and stand up slowly as the heat sometimes causes dizziness.

   b) Take a long, hot shower and aim the full force of the water at the painful joint(s). Hand-held showers with a massage unit can be pleasant.

   c) An electric heating pad can be placed over the affected area. Be sure the hot pad has a cover and that you do not fall asleep with it plugged in. It is best not to lie directly on the pad, and never use an electric pad with anything wet.

   d) Fill a hot-water bottle with hot water. Be sure it is not hot enough to burn you. Again, it is best not to lie directly on the water bottle.

   e) Stand next to your heater or radiator.

5. If you don't get good results from heat, the application of cold may prove more effective, especially for the "hot" joint of rheumatoid arthritis. Cold relaxes muscles and produces a numbing effect, thus decreasing pain and increasing joint motion. As with heat, there are a few important principles of application:

   a) If you are especially sensitive to cold or have decreased sensation or circulation such as in Raynaud's Disease or vasculitis, do not apply cold. Ask your doctor or therapist if you are unsure.

   b) Apply just long enough to achieve a numbing effect—no more than 15 to 20 minutes.

c) Be cautious when exercising after applying cold; the numbing effect may allow you to overdo. Remember, if the joint is "hot," restrict exercise to moving the joint through its full range of motion twice a day.

d) Place the cold pack over the joint, not between the joint and a firm surface.

e) Check during and after application for any sign of a break in the skin.

Cold packs can be bought, or you can create your own. Wrapping the pack in a warm, moist towel will help you adjust to the cold. Use whichever cold pack method is easiest and most effective for you:

a) Several resourceful people have suggested a sack of frozen peas! You can refreeze it and use it again.

b) Massage with a large ice cube.

c) Make a slush pack: Line a bowl with two heavy plastic bags; fill with three cups water and one cup denatured alcohol. Fasten the bags and place the bowl in the freezer until slush forms. You can refreeze a slush pack.

How Should I Exercise?

Be consistent and stick to your chosen set of exercises. Begin at a comfortable level for you and gradually increase the number of repetitions. Progress more slowly with rheumatoid joints that are prone to "hot" periods. With this gradual progression you will avoid unnecessary pain.

Your exercises should minimize stress on the affected joints. Carefully assess the stress each exercise imposes on the priority joint and those surrounding it. You will find further discussion of this throughout the chapter.

Exercises for arthritis should be performed with a slow, steady rhythm. Give your muscles time to relax between repetitions of each exercise (10 to 15 seconds). After a muscle is used, it must relax and lengthen so that waste products of muscle action can be carried away. Learning to relax readily and completely during exercise will make any exercise program more effective and enjoyable. Techniques aimed at release of residual tension throughout the body will be discussed in Chapter 8.

It is important to coordinate your breathing with exercise. Breathe deeply and rhythmically as you exercise; never hold your breath. Interspersing deep breathing with exercise ensures an adequate oxygen supply to working muscles as well as release of tension. Deep breathing involves inhaling slowly and gently through your nose and drawing air down into your abdomen. Hold for at least five counts. Exhale slowly and gently through lightly closed lips for at least five counts. You can do this breathing exercise in between the exercises described later.

What Should I Avoid?

Remember that your exercises should minimize stress on the joints. Avoid high-tension exercises such as weight lifting. If your weight-bearing joints are affected (hips, knees, ankles, or spine), jogging should be approached cautiously. Bicycling for a painful knee should also be approached with caution: set a stationary bicycle on the lowest resistance or use a low gear on a conventional bicycle.

If a chosen exercise for one joint places excessive stress on another involved joint—for example, a shoulder exercise that stresses an involved hand, or a hip exercise that stresses a painful low back—modify the exercise or substitute another.

As stated earlier, avoid exercising the hot, inflamed joint, but remember to move it through its full range of motion twice a day. Deep massage of the painful joint should also be avoided. Never take extra medication to mask joint pain before exercising. This could result in joint damage, as pain is your real guide to when you've done too much.

Since warmth helps relax stiff muscles and joints, avoid becoming chilled during exercise. Wear warm clothing and do not exercise in a draft or a cold room. Hand exercises can be done in a basin of warm water.

When Have I Done Too Much?

Use common sense and listen to the signals your body gives you. A general rule of thumb is that if exercise-induced pain lasts longer than two hours, cut back. Do not stop. The key here is "exercise-induced." If you do your exercises and then go out and garden for three hours the chances are that the prolonged gardening is responsible for any residual pain.

Any exercise program is bound to have setbacks, but these are not permanent. If you experience exercise-induced pain for longer than two hours, decrease the number of repetitions or be less forceful. If that does not help, choose a different exercise that will achieve the same result but that is more appropriate for you. Also, review the principles of exercise discussed here and in the sections on stretching and strengthening exercises.

TYPES OF EXERCISE

There are three basic types of exercise. **Range-of-motion** or **stretching exercises** involve moving a joint as far as it will comfortably go (through its full range of motion) and then coaxing it a little farther, just past the point of beginning pain or discomfort. These exercises are designed to increase and then maintain joint mobility, thus decreasing pain and improving function.

Strengthening exercises increase muscle strength and thus lend stability to vulnerable joints. They improve your ability to bear weight, lift objects, and sustain movement. Strengthening exercises should be done in such a way as to minimize stress on the joints. For this reason, good strengthening exercises are *isometric*. These exercises involve use (contraction) of a muscle or muscles without movement at the joint. Discussion and examples of the isometric principle can be found in the section on specific strengthening exercises. Remember, strengthening exercises are not a substitute for stretching exercises. They will not increase joint range of motion.

Endurance exercises are necessary because neither stretching nor strengthening exercises will increase your endurance. More dynamic forms of exercise, such as walking, swimming, bicycling, jogging, dancing, or cross-country skiing will promote cardiovascular fitness. Include some kind of dynamic exercise in your program every day, but remember to start out easy and progress slowly. To help reduce stress while walking or dancing wear low-heeled, rubber-soled, lightweight shoes. A good running shoe is essential for any runner with joint or muscle problems; try them on before you buy and consult a running guide for current recommendations. These are often excellent shoes for just walking.

STRETCHING OR RANGE-OF-MOTION EXERCISES

The general rule for stretching exercises is to move the joint as far as it will comfortably go (its full range of motion) and then coax it a little further, just past the point of first pain. Do not "bounce." A gentle, sustained stretch will be less stressful to your joints and more effective. **Each stretching exercise should be repeated three to ten times, two to four times a day, depending on pain.** Remember one of the basic principles of exercise as you decide on the number of repetitions—start slow and easy. If you have exercise-induced pain lasting longer than two hours, cut back a little. Don't give up.

The exercises in this section are examples of stretching exercises. As you become familiar with the principles involved, you may want to design your own exercises or incorporate others you have learned.

Before proceeding to the exercises, take a mental survey of your joints. To maintain your present function, you must move every joint in your body through its full range of motion every day. This movement usually occurs during your daily activities. However, because of your arthritis you may be protecting some joints by not moving them. Do you have joints that are not moved through their full range of motion every day or joints that you cannot move as far as you used to? If so, please list them here.

1.

2.

3.

4.

5.

It is difficult to stretch more than two or three joints at a time. Choose two or three priority joints with which to start working and pick a goal for each joint. For example:

1. Shoulder. I want to reach above my head to touch the top shelf.

2. Fingers. I want to touch the tips of my fingers to my palm.

MY PRIORITY JOINTS   *MY GOAL*

1.

2.

3.

Once you have reached your goal for one of these joints, you can then add stretching exercises for another. But remember, to maintain the mobility that you worked so hard to achieve you must move that joint through its full range of motion once or twice a day. If you notice that you are losing ground with that joint, then resume a more concentrated stretching program.

Now, turn to the appropriate stretching exercises for your priority joints.

HANDS

The hand is a very delicate and intricate part of the body. The following exercises will help maintain or increase movements essential to the skilled movements we perform with our hands. If you have severe hand deformity or involvement you may wish to consult an occupational or physical therapist in developing your initial program. Also, when choosing exercises for other parts of the body, remember to assess the stress imposed on the hands and modify the exercise if necessary. See Chapter 6 for suggestions on how to modify activities to protect the involved hand.

1. One-Two-Three Finger Exercise

For optimum function you should be able to touch the tips of your fingers to the palm. When stretching the fingertips toward the palm use the "one-two-three" approach. Begin with the joint closest to the tip of the finger (A), then move on to the middle joint (B). When your fingertips are touching the palm or as close as possible, bend the knuckle joint (C). You may exercise your

fingers individually or together, using your other hand to guide the movement
if necessary.

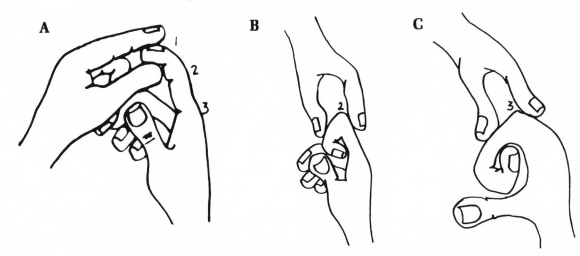

2. Three-Two-One Finger Exercise

If any of the joints in your fingers will not straighten completely, try this
exercise, which is the reverse of 1. With you fingertips as close to the palm as
possible, begin to uncurl your hand. Begin with the knuckle joint (A), move to
the middle joint (B), and finally exercise the joint closest to the tip of the
finger (C).

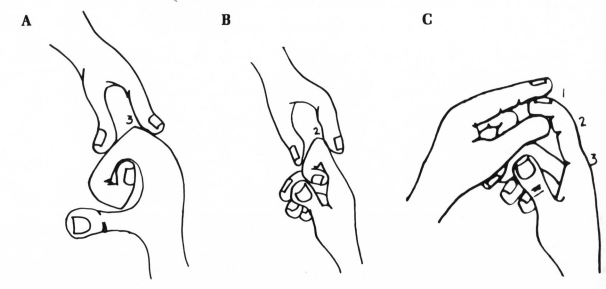

3. Fingers Flat Exercise

This is another exercise for straightening the joints of the fingers. Lay your hand as flat as possible on a table. Place the heel of your other hand across your fingers and gently press down, straightening the fingers.

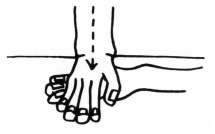

4. The Thumb Walk

Try to form a letter "O" with each attempt of this exercise. Lightly touch the tip of the thumb to the tip of the index finger (A), then spread your fingers as wide as you can (B). Proceed on to touch the tip of the thumb to the tips of your other fingers, spreading the fingers wide after each attempt. If you cannot quite bring the thumb to touch the finger, use the other hand to coax them closer together.

A   B

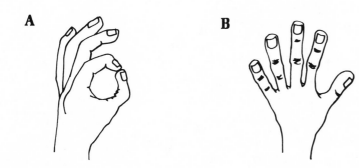

WRISTS

The next two exercises will help maintain or improve your ability to move the wrist back and forth.

5. The Palm Press

First, place your hands together, palms touching and fingers straight (A). Press the right hand backward with the left hand (B), then reverse and press the left hand backward with the right hand. Exert pressure at the palm, *not* the fingertips. Coax the hand just past the point of discomfort.

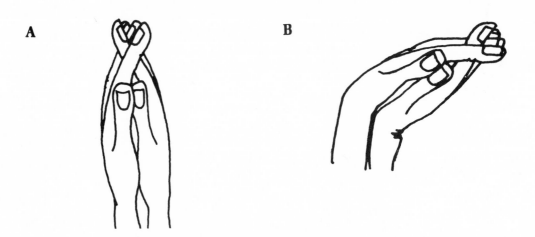

6. Wrist Table Stretch

For a more vigorous wrist stretch hang the hand over the edge of a table or arm rest with the palm down. Raise the hand up as far as possible, using your other hand to assist with the stretch (A). Then lower the hand, stretching just past the point of discomfort (B).

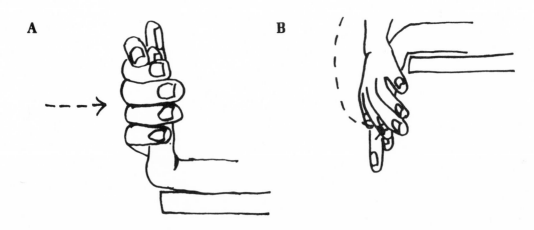

7. The Slide

If you notice that your fingers drift toward the little finger side of the hand (a common deformity in rheumatoid arthritis), this exercise is for you. Place your forearm on a table, palm down. Slide each finger toward the thumb, not moving the forearm. Use your other hand to assist if necessary. Repeat with the other hand. The exercise works to keep your knuckles and wrist in correct alignment with your forearm, promoting optimal function.

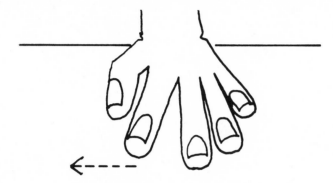

8. The Door Opener

This is an exercise to stretch the muscles and ligaments that rotate the forearm, allowing you to turn doorknobs and unlock doors. Start with your forearm resting on a table, palm down. Turn your hand so the palm faces up (A). If you use your other hand to assist with the stretch, grasp the lower part of the forearm, *not* the hand.

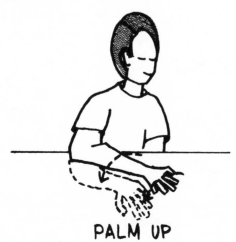

PALM UP

ELBOWS

9. The Elbow Chop

The diagonal pattern in this exercise is similar to that of chopping wood and is designed to help you bend and straighten the elbow completely. Place hands together and bend both elbows until your hands touch your right shoulder (A). Then bring hands down to touch the left knee, straightening elbows completely (B). Remember to coax the elbow a little farther than it wants to go. Reverse directions, going from left shoulder to right knee.

A

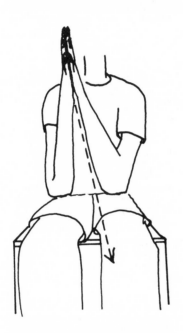

B

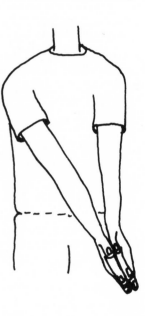

SHOULDERS

The shoulder is one of those joints that moves in many directions. When choosing stretching exercises, it is important to decide which functions are most important to you.

10. The Pendulum

This exercise is good as the beginning exercise for the very painful or limited shoulder. It facilitates relaxation of the shoulder muscles as well as free joint movement in all directions. From a standing or sitting position, lean slightly forward. Let your arm hang freely in front of you. Relax and feel the weight of your arm. Keeping the arm straight, begin with small circles and gradually increase their size. Remember to exercise to just past the point of discomfort. Don't get carried away with your circles.

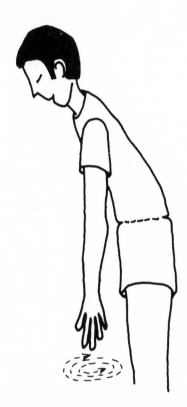

11. The Shoulder Rotator

If you have difficulty touching the back of your neck, combing your hair, or zipping a back zipper, then you probably need to work on outward rotation of the shoulder. Here are two ways to accomplish this movement. (A) Clasp your hands together at the back of your neck and pull the elbows as far back as possible. You should feel a stretch at the front of the shoulder and chest. (B) If you are not yet ready for the first exercise, begin with this method.

Hold your arm close to your side with elbow bent. Keeping elbow at your side, rotate hand and forearm outward as far away from your stomach as possible. You may use your other hand to assist with the stretch.

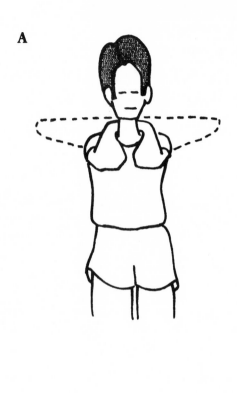

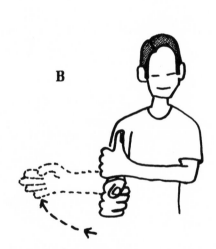

Here are three exercises to increase your ability to reach overhead. This is important for dressing, getting things off shelves, or picking apples. You do not need to do all of these exercises. One exercise repeated three to ten times, two to four times a day, is sufficient. Pick the one that suits you best, or change exercises occasionally for variety.

12. The Shoulder Cradle

If your shoulder is still very painful, this exercise may be better tolerated. With your arm supported at the elbow by the opposite hand (A), raise the arm up over your head. You can rest your forearm on your head as you coax your shoulder just past the point of pain (B). This exercise may be easier lying down.

A

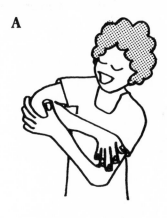

B

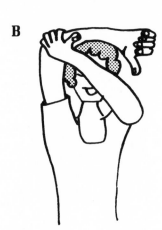

13. The Wand Exercise

Use a cane, yardstick, or mop handle as your wand. Place one hand on each end and raise the wand as high overhead as possible. You might try doing this in front of a mirror. You don't have to move both ends to the same height —play around with it. If holding the wand causes pain in your hand, try building up the grip area as described in Chapter 6 (Principle 8b).

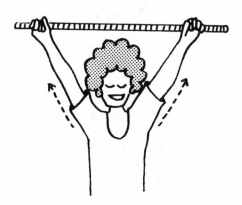

14. The Shoulder Pulley

Throw a piece of rope over the top of an open door, creating a modified pulley system. Hold one end of the rope in each hand. As you pull down on one end, the other arm will be raised up. Coax the arm a little higher than it wants to go and then pull down, raising the opposite arm.

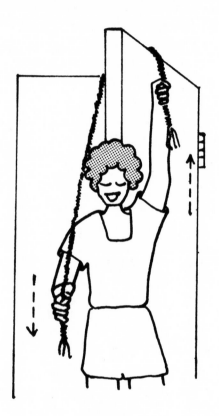

HIPS

The hip is the largest joint of the body and like the shoulder can move in several directions. In choosing which exercise to do, decide which movements are most limited or painful and concentrate on them initially. You should do the selected exercises three to ten times, two to four times a day. Stretch just past the point of pain. If exercise-induced pain persists for longer than two hours after exercise, you are doing too much. *Do not stop, just cut back.*

15. The Spread Eagle

This exercise increases hip motion to the side, which is necessary for riding a bicycle, getting in and out of a car, or riding a horse. Lie on your back. Spread your legs as far apart as possible and then coax them a little farther. You might want someone to measure the distance between your knees so you can keep track of your progress. If this is difficult or if you feel discomfort in your lower back, move one leg at a time while keeping the other leg bent.

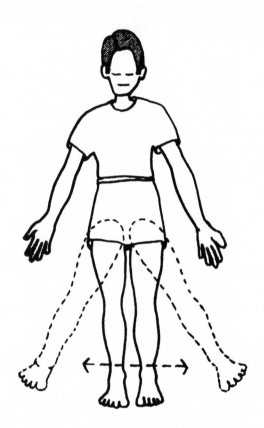

16. Knee-to-Chest

This exercise will help increase the hip motion forward, which is important for activities such as walking, climbing stairs, and getting on and off low furniture. Lie on your back. Keep one leg straight and bring your other knee toward your chest. You can place your hands under the thigh to assist with the stretch. This exercise also helps to stretch the low back. You may want to begin with your other leg slightly bent to decrease strain on the low back.

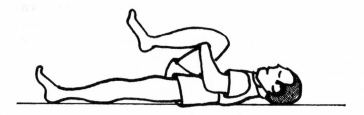

17. The Back Kick

This exercise is designed to increase the backward motion of the hip, which is important for walking, running, and cross-country skiing. From a standing position, hold on to a counter for support and move the leg up and back, knee straight. Start gently and keep your hips facing forward.

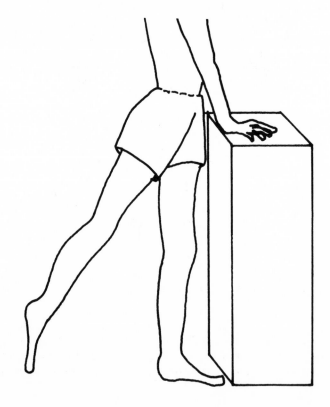

18. The Leg Lift

If you cannot stand up to do the Back Kick, this exercise also helps to increase the backward motion of the hip. Lie face down. This alone may provide a good stretch for those who spend a great deal of time sitting or in bed. If this position is comfortable, raise your leg as high as possible. This exercise should not be done by people with low back or disc problems.

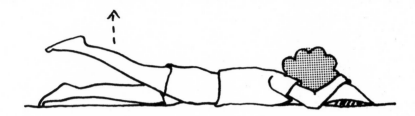

19. The Hip Rotator

This exercise increases the ability of the hip to rotate (roll in and out). This is important for activities such as dancing or rolling over and getting out of bed. Lie on your back, hands out to the side or behind your head. Bend your hips and knees and place feet flat. Cross your right leg over the left knee (A). Rotate hips to the right, trying to touch the knee to the floor (B). Keep your upper body flat on the floor. Repeat to the other side. This is also a good exercise for stretching the low and middle back, but some may find it too strenuous for the back.

A

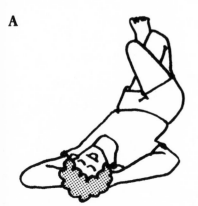

B

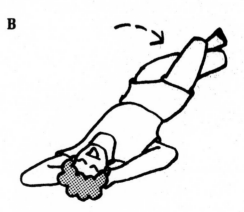

KNEES

The knee is subject to a lot of stress due to its weight-bearing duties and limited muscular support. When stretching the knee it is important to minimize the stress on the joint. Thus you should not be standing when you exercise your knees as the weight of your body adds stress.

The next two exercises are designed to increase your ability to bend and straighten the knee, which is important for climbing stairs or getting up and down from a chair, and most important for standing and walking without fatigue.

20. Knee Bend 1

Lie on your back with both knees bent, feet flat. Bring your knee toward your chest. Using your hands to assist, gently bend the knee, trying to touch your heel to your buttock.

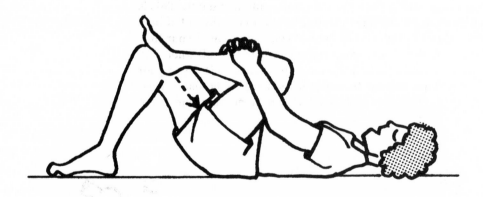

21. Knee Bend 2

If exercise 20 doesn't suit you, try this one. Sit on a straight-backed chair and bend your knee as far back as possible. (Be sure that it is not a part of the chair that keeps you from going farther). To get an extra stretch, place your hands on the side of the chair and scoot forward toward the edge, keeping your feet in the same position.

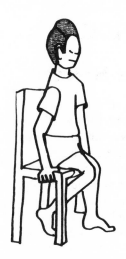

22. The Knee Straightener

The ability to straighten the knee is very important for walking or any standing activity. When one spends a lot of time sitting, the muscles and ligaments in the back of the knee tend to tighten, making it difficult to completely straighten the knee. This exercise is designed to stretch these tissues with a minimum of stress on the joints. Sitting in a straight-backed chair, place your foot on a chair or high footstool. Bend the knee slightly and then straighten by pushing the back of the knee toward the floor. If you find this easy, add another stretch. Place the support. Carefully lean forward; keep your back straight. You will feel a stretch along the hamstring muscles on the back of your leg.

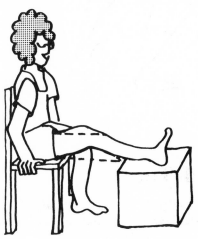

ANKLES AND FEET

23. The Achilles Stretch

This exercise is designed to stretch your Achilles tendon, which is the large tendon you feel at the back of your ankle. It is important to maintain flexibility in this tendon for standing and walking. Joggers should be sure to stretch this tendon before starting out.

Stand at the end of a table and hold onto the sides. Bend the knee of the leg you are not stretching so it almost touches the table. Put the leg to be stretched behind you, keeping both feet flat on the floor. Now lean forward, keeping your back knee straight. You should feel a good stretch in the calf of the leg. This exercise can also be done leaning against a wall or fence.

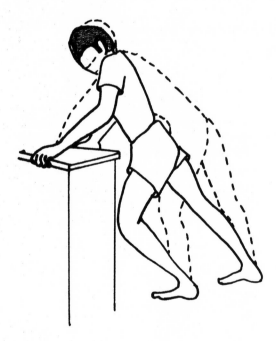

24. The Heel-Toe

Sit in a chair or on the edge of the bed with both feet flat on the floor. First, raise your toes and forefeet as high as you can, keeping your heels on the floor (A). Then, keep your toes on the floor and raise your heels as high as you can (B). This stretches tendons, calf muscles, and the ankle joints.

A

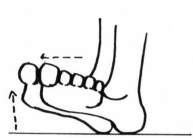

B

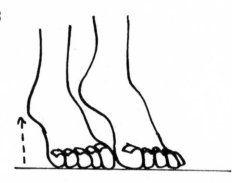

25. The Heel-Toe Dance

Sit in a chair with your feet flat on the ground. With heels on the floor, lift feet and toes as high as you can (A). Keeping the heels on the floor, move feet and toes to the right (B). Then come up on your toes as high as you can and move your heels to the right (C). Reverse and walk feet to the left in the same manner. This helps the rotation at the ankle.

A

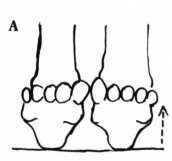

B

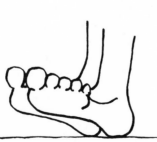

C

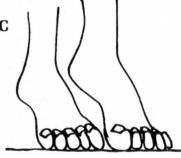

26. The Foot Roll

Place a dowel (large mop handle, closet rod, rolling pin) under the arch of the foot and roll it back and forth. This feels great and it stretches the ligaments of the arch of the foot.

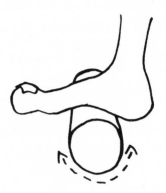

NECK

The neck involves many joints that work together to allow movement. It is one of the easiest parts of the body to exercise. However, it is important to be gentle when you exercise the neck. If you have learned to do neck exercises using circular motions, be sure you only make a half-circle in each direction. A complete circle may cause severe pain for people with bone spurs or a disc problem. If you have found circular exercises to be unsatisfactory, the following exercises should be more appropriate, and we prefer them.

If your neck pain is a new occurrence and the pain is moderate to severe, if you have pain that radiates down your arm with neck movement, or if numbness, tingling, or marked weakness are present in the arm, you should consult your physician or physical therapist before proceeding with these exercises.

27. The Three-Way Neck Stretch

1. Relax and slowly drop your chin to your chest, then slowly raise your head and very gently drop the head backward. Do not proceed with this

exercise if you feel a sharp pain or pain down your arm. Return head to the upright position slowly. This motion should never be forced.

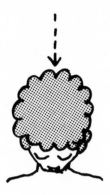 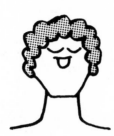

2. Turn to look over your right shoulder, then turn to look as far over the left shoulder as possible.

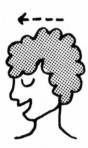 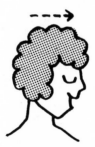

3. Tilt your head to the right and then to the left. Try to touch your ear to your shoulder.

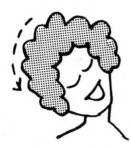 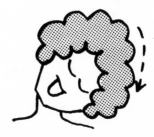

BACK

The following are a series of exercises for those with chronic back problems, especially those with ankylosing spondylitis or generalized stiffness. If your back pain is a new occurrence and the pain is moderate to severe, you should consult your physician or physical therapist before proceeding with these exercises. Also, if you notice pain that radiates down your leg, numbness, tingling, or marked weakness, consult a physician. If exercise-induced pain lasts longer than two hours, cut back a little. Those with ankylosing spondylitis will want to do deep-breathing exercises in addition to ensure good mobility of the rib cage.

28. The Pelvic Tilt

This exercise should be the beginning point for the person with low back problems. Lie on the bed or floor with both knees bent, feet flat. Place your hands on your abdomen. Flatten the small of your back against the floor by tightening your buttocks and pulling in your stomach. If this concept is difficult for you, think of bringing your pubic bone toward your chin. Once you have mastered the pelvic tilt in the lying position, try it while standing and sitting.

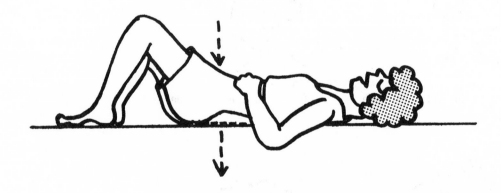

29. Knee-to-Chin Stretch

For a nice low back stretch, lie on the floor with knees bent, feet flat. Bring one knee toward your chin, using your hands to assist with the stretch. Maintain this position for five seconds and lower the leg slowly. Repeat with the other knee. To stretch the upper and middle back at the same time, raise your head and shoulder from the floor as you bring your knee toward your chin. If this creates or increases neck pain, discontinue this portion of the exercise.

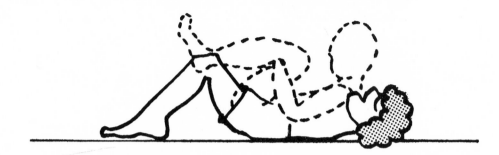

30. The Low Back Rock

Lie on your back with your knees bent and feet flat. Pull knees up to chest, one at a time, grasping under the thighs to assist with the stretch. Rest in this position for five seconds, then gently rock knees from one side to the other, keeping upper back and shoulders on the floor.

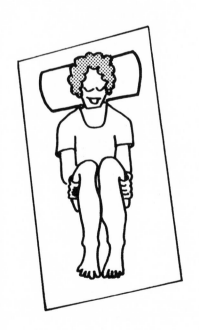 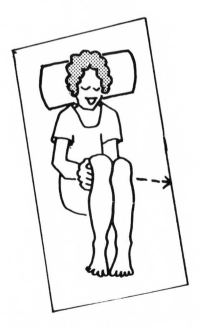

31. The Shoulder-Blade Pinch

This is a good exercise for the middle and upper back. Sit on the edge of a bed or chair. Pinch your shoulder blades together by moving your elbows as far back as possible.

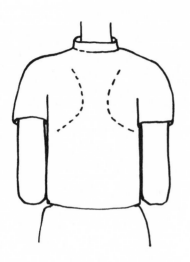 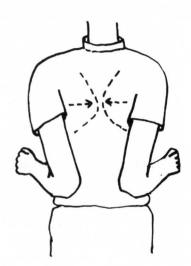

32. The Back Lift

Another way to improve flexibility of the spine is to lie on your stomach. Raise up onto your forearms. If you feel no discomfort, raise up onto extended arms. This exercise should be avoided by people with moderate to severe low back pain.

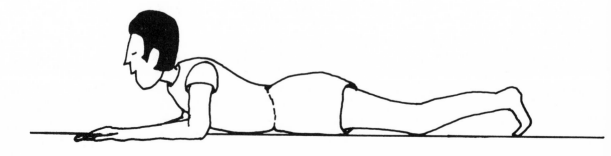

33. The Cat

This exercise should not be done by persons with severe knee, ankle, or hand problems because it places stress on these joints. Assume a crawling position on all fours, with knees bent, arms straight. Taking a deep breath, arch your back as a frightened cat does. Then slowly drop the arch, exhaling completely.

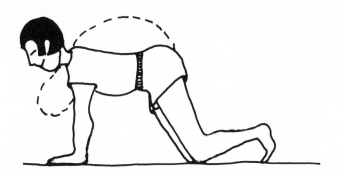

STRENGTHENING EXERCISES

The purpose of these exercises is to maintain strong muscles and to strengthen muscles with as little stress on the joints as possible. Many of them are examples of isometric exercise. If you understand the principles of isometric exercise, you can devise your own exercise for any muscle group. These exercises will not maintain or increase joint mobility.

As described earlier, isometric exercise involves use (contraction) of a muscle with no movement of the joint. One way to accomplish this is to use the muscle to pull or push against a stationary object. The stationary object may be anything from a wall to a body part to an exercise belt. For example, place your hand on the wall and push. You can feel the muscles in your arm working; however, no movement of the joints is taking place. This is an isometric exercise. Here's another example: Sit in a chair and place your right hand on your right knee. Press your right knee against the hand, allowing no movement of the arm or leg. You have used another body part as the stationary object.

One nice thing about isometric exercises is that you do not have to do many to receive the benefits. Each exercise, held for a count of six seconds, three to four times a day, is sufficient. *Gradually* tense and relax the muscle, avoiding sudden, quick movement. To prevent the tendency to hold your breath, count the six seconds out loud. If exercise-induced pain lasts longer than two hours, cut back a little. As with the famous tortoise, slow and steady wins the race. Long, sustained isometric exercise is not advisable for heart patients, but the following exercises should not be harmful. If in doubt, consult your physician.

For these exercises you will need an exercise belt of some kind. It is best if this belt has some give to it. The inner tube from a bicycle tire, a bungie cord (holds packages on bicycles), or a strong stretch belt will do fine. If all else fails, a regular leather belt will suffice. The exercise belt is a closed loop, 30 to 48 inches in circumference.

Before proceeding to specific exercises, take a mental inventory of your body. Are there parts of your body you would like to strengthen? If so, define which parts.

1.

2.

3.

4.

5.

Now pick two or three priorities and proceed to the section dealing with your priority areas. Remember, your goal is not to do every strengthening exercise in the book but to use the ones you specifically need.

1.

2.

3.

HANDS

34. The Finger Press

To strengthen the muscles that bend the fingers and help you pick up objects, try this exercise. Lightly press the tip of the thumb to the tip of the index finger. Hold for six seconds, maintaining a perfect "O" shape, then relax. Continue, lightly pressing the tip of the thumb to the tip of each finger. To help maintain the "O" shape, place a pill bottle or other cylinder in your hand. Those with rheumatoid arthritis should not press the fingers together but just touch them lightly.

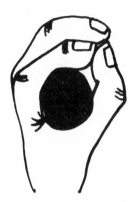

35. The Finger Lift

To strengthen the muscles that straighten the fingers, lay your hand flat on a table. Lay your other hand across the fingers to be exercised. Lift the fingers of the bottom hand, pushing against the top hand. Hold for six seconds; relax. If you have significant weakness, do each finger separately. You should exert only gentle pressure for this exercise.

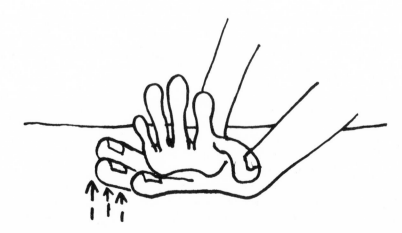

36. The Finger Slide

Place your hand flat, fingers spread, on the table. Lift and slide each finger toward the thumb. Resist slightly with the other hand. This will help prevent drifting of the fingers toward the little-finger side of the hand.

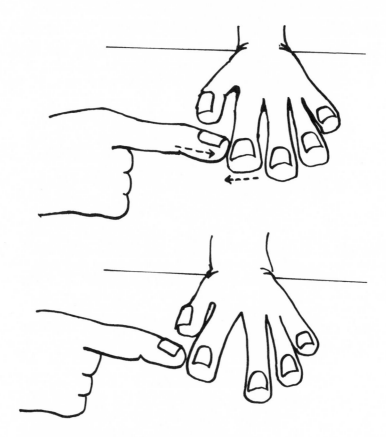

WRISTS

37. The Wrist Press

This exercise will strengthen the muscles that bend and straighten the wrist. Rest your hand on a table or armrest. Place the heel of the other hand on top. Raise the bottom hand, pushing against the top hand. Hold for six seconds, then relax. Reverse positions of the hand and repeat. Remember, while you are pressing the hands together, allow no joint movement. If it is painful to use your other hand as the stationary object, try to lift the hand against another stable object, such as the chair arm.

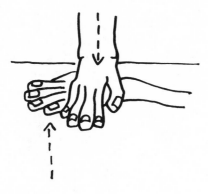

ELBOWS

38. The Biceps Bulge

This will strengthen the muscles that bend and straighten the elbow. Place your exercise belt slightly above each wrist, palms facing up. Bend one elbow and straighten the other, pulling the belt tight. Hold for six seconds. Relax. Reverse arm positions. If you do not have an exercise belt, cross your forearms, palms up, and press together. Hold for six seconds. Relax and reverse arm positions.

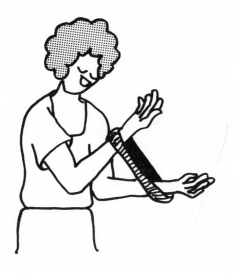

SHOULDERS
39. The Side Pull

Place the exercise belt around your forearms. With the elbows straight, palms facing each other, move your arms out to the side until the belt is tight. Hold for six seconds. Relax. If you do not have an exercise belt, perform the same movement, pushing against a wall, door frame, or some other stationary object.

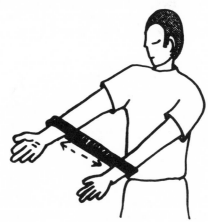

40. The Robot

This exercise will strengthen the muscles that raise and lower your arm. Place the exercise belt around your forearms, palms down. Keeping elbows straight, pull up with one arm and down with the other until the belt is tight. Hold for six seconds, then relax. Reverse arm positions and repeat. If you do not have an exercise belt, perform the same movement using a table, wall, or your other forearm as the stationary object.

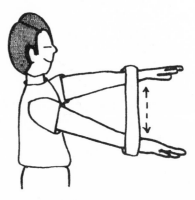

41. The Bow and Arrow

This is a fun exercise for strengthening many of the arm muscles. Hold the exercise belt in both hands. Push out to the side with one arm and pull back with the other, as if shooting a bow and arrow or a giant rubber band. Hold for six seconds, then relax. Reverse arm positions. Those with hand involvement should modify this exercise because gripping the belt causes stress. Be creative!

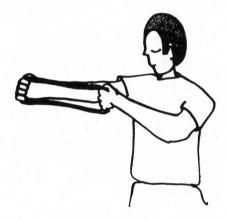

HIPS

42. The "Cheek to Cheek"

This exercise will strengthen the muscles that move your leg backward. Squeeze the buttocks tightly together. Hold for six seconds. Relax. This exercise may be done while lying down, sitting, or standing.

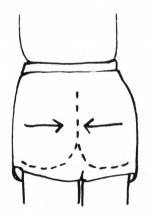

43. The Leg Spreader

The muscles that move your legs out to the side must be strong if you are to walk well. Lie on your back, with the exercise belt placed around your ankles. (If your knees are painful place the belt above the knees.) Spread your legs apart until the exercise belt is as tight as possible. Hold for six seconds, then relax. Do not let your foot roll in or out. You may do each leg separately if you wish.

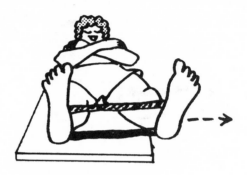

44. The Straight-Leg Raise

This familiar old exercise will strengthen the muscles that bend the hip as well as the muscle that runs across the front of the knee. Lie on your back, arms in a comfortable position. Tighten the muscle that runs across the front of the knee and then raise your leg one to two feet off the ground, keeping the knee straight. Do not arch your back. Hold for six seconds. Relax. If you have low back discomfort you should do this exercise with the other knee bent. As your muscles become stronger, place the exercise belt around your ankles and perform the same exercise. Pull the belt tight, hold for six seconds, and then lower the leg slowly.

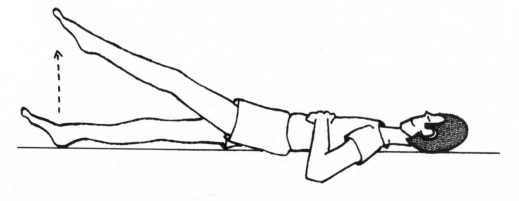

KNEES

45. The Quad Set

This is a good place for the person with very weak or painful knees to start. The exercise will strengthen the muscles that straighten the knee. These muscles are crucial for walking, going up and down stairs, or getting out of low furniture. Sit with your back supported, legs stretched out in front of you. (You may bend one knee if this is more comfortable.) Tighten the muscle that runs across the front of the knee by pulling your toes toward your head and pushing the back of the knee down into the bed or floor. Hold for six seconds. Relax. If sitting is difficult, this exercise may be done while lying down.

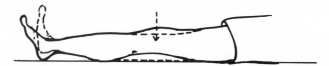

46. The Knee Scissor

Here's another exercise to strengthen the muscles that straighten the knee. It will also strengthen the muscles that bend the knee. Sit in a straight-backed chair. Place the exercise belt around both ankles. Straighten one knee while you pull back with the other until the belt is very tight. Hold for six seconds. Relax. To reduce stress on the knee joint, lean back slightly as you do this exercise.

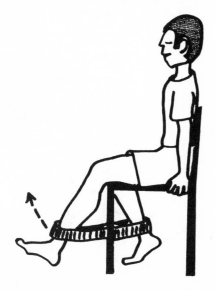

47. The Heel Press

To strengthen the muscles at the back of the thigh that bend the knee, sit in a straight-backed chair. Bend the knee, pressing the heel against the leg of the chair. Hold for six seconds. Relax.

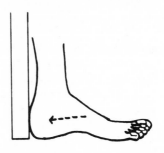

ANKLES AND FEET

48. The Tiptoe

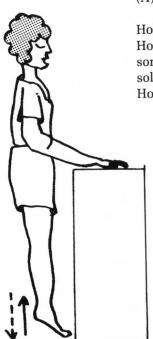

Holding on lightly to a counter or table for support, raise up on your tiptoes (A).

Holding on lightly to a counter or table for support, raise up on your tiptoes (A). Hold for six seconds. Lower slowly. This exercise may be too stressful for some, especially if you are overweight. As an alternate exercise, place the sole of your foot against a stationary object (wall, chair leg) and push (B). Hold for six seconds; relax.

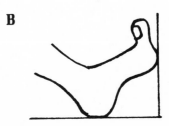

NECK

If your neck pain is a new occurrence and the pain is moderate to severe, if you have pain that radiates down your arm with neck movement, or if numbness, tingling, or marked weakness are present in the arm, consult a physician or physical therapist before proceeding with these exercises.

49. The Head Press

Here is an easy way to strengthen the muscles that bend and straighten the neck. Place your forearm against your forehead and press with your head. Hold for six seconds, allowing no movement. Relax. Then place your forearm on the back of the head and push. Hold for six seconds. Relax. If you cannot use your arm as the stationary object, a wall or a car headrest will do just as well.

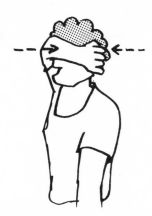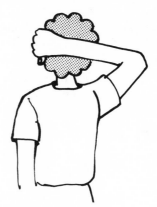

50. The Neck Strengthener

The same muscles can be strengthened while lying in bed. Lift your head up off the pillow. Hold for six seconds, then relax. Press your head down into the pillow. Hold for six seconds, then relax. If lifting your head is painful, press against your forearm as in exercise 49.

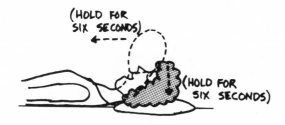

(HOLD FOR SIX SECONDS)

(HOLD FOR SIX SECONDS)

BACK AND STOMACH

If your back pain is a new occurrence and the pain is moderate to severe, if pain radiates down your leg or around to the chest, or if numbness, tingling, or marked weakness exist, consult a physician or physical therapist before proceeding.

Firm stomach and back muscles are important to provide the support necessary for an erect posture and to avoid back strain. In addition to the following exercises, the Pelvic Tilt (exercise 28) is helpful and should be done frequently during the day, in any position.

51. The Partial Sit-Up

It is not necessary to do a full sit-up to exercise the stomach muscles. A partial sit-up will place less stress on the joints and is sufficient. Lie on your back on a firm surface, knees bent, feet flat. Raise your head and shoulders as far off the surface as possible. Hold for six seconds, then lower slowly. Breathe out as you raise your body, count to six out loud as you hold, and breathe in as you lower your body. *Do not hold your breath.* If your neck is painful during this exercise, try the next one instead. Don't cheat by tucking your feet under a chair!

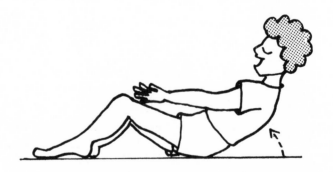

52. The Back Sit

This is a fun alternative to the sit-up and is easier on the neck. Sit upright on a firm surface. Lean partially backward, hold for six seconds, then return to sitting. As your stomach muscles strengthen you should be able to lean farther and farther backward. Breathe out as you lean back, count to six out loud as you hold, and breathe in as you return to sitting.

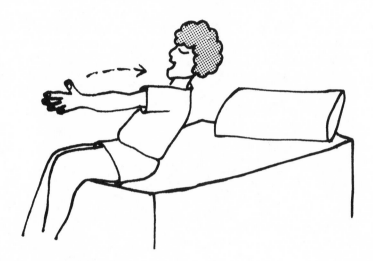

53. The Back Push

To strengthen the muscles that straighten the back, sit in a straight-backed chair or against the wall. Push your shoulders and shoulder blades into the chair or wall. Hold for six seconds. Relax. You will feel the stomach muscles tighten as well; the stomach muscles help support the back.

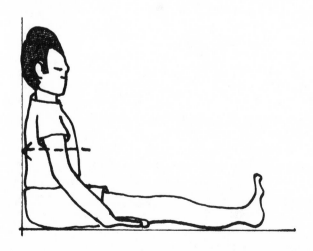

54. The Back Lift

This exercise will also strengthen the muscles that straighten the back, but i
is more strenuous. Lie on your stomach, arms at your sides. Lift your head
shoulders, and arms up off the floor or bed. Hold for six seconds. Relax. I
this does not feel too stressful, try lifting your legs off the floor at the same
time. This is generally not a good exercise for the person with moderate to
severe low back pain but is beneficial for the person with general stiffness or
ankylosing spondylitis.

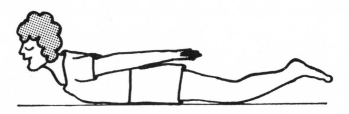

A MATTER OF PRINCIPLE: EXERCISE REVIEW

Let's go back over the critical points. The two most important kinds o
exercise to maintain and improve the function of arthritic joints and sur
rounding muscles are:

1. **Stretching exercises** to maintain and increase joint mobility and thus
    function. They should be performed three to ten times a session, two to
    four times a day, depending on pain.

2. **Strengthening exercises** to increase muscle strength and improve the
    ability to bear weight, lift objects, and sustain movement. Usually, iso
    metric exercises are best. Hold each exercise for six seconds and repea
    three to four times once a day.

Endurance and relaxation activities should also be a part of your daily
schedule to provide for a well-rounded exercise program. Balance you
exercise activities with times of rest during the day. You can combine res
periods with relaxation training. Also remember that is is important to
prepare for exercise by warming up.

Design your own exercise program to meet your special needs. Asses
each exercise for its benefit to your priority joints and for any excessive stres
on other involved joints. Begin slowly and build your program according to
your response to the exercise. If at any time exercise-induced pain continue
for more than two hours after exercise, you are doing too much. Do not stop
exercising, but cut back a little. Remember, if you have a hot joint, restrai
yourself to moving the joint through its full range of motion twice a day.

A MATTER OF PROGRAM: SETTING UP YOUR OWN EXERCISE PROGRAM

Now that you have chosen specific exercises, it may be helpful to write out your exercise program and keep an exercise diary. This tends to help you get started, and when you look back on it, it will show you how far you have progressed.

GUIDELINES

The following will give you some guidelines for setting up your exercise program. Read these guidelines carefully and use them as you plan your program.

Stretching Exercises (Exercises 1-33)

1. Start doing three repetitions of each exercise twice a day.

2. If for four days you have no exercise-induced pain lasting longer than two hours, add two repetitions (five in all) and do the exercises three times a day.

3. If no exercise-induced pain lasting longer than two hours is present in an additional four-day period, add two more repetitions (seven in all) and do the exercises four times a day.

4. If in the next four days you have no exercise-induced pain lasting longer than two hours, add three more repetitions (ten in all) and do the exercises four times a day.

5. If exercise-induced pain continues for more than two hours after exercise, cut back to the next lowest level and continue at that level for four days, then try the next highest level again.

6. If exercise-induced pain lasting longer than two hours occurs at the first level, try not to stretch so far (just past the point of pain). If pain still persists, cut back to two repetitions once a day or choose a different exercise that will achieve the same result.

7. Once you have reached your goal for a joint, remember to move it through its maximal range at least once or twice a day. This will ensure that you maintain the mobility that you worked so hard to obtain. If you notice that you are losing ground with that joint, then resume a more concentrated exercise program.

Strengthening Exercises (Exercises 34-54)

1. Start doing each exercise twice, once a day.

2. If no exercise-induced pain lasting longer than two hours occurs in a four-day period, add one repetition (three in all).

3. If no exercise-induced pain occurs for four more days, add one repetition (four in all).

4. If exercise-induced pain continues for more than two hours after exercise, cut back to the next lowest level and continue at that level for four days, then try to move to the next highest level again.

5. If pain occurs at the first level, reduce the force of your exercise. If pain still persists, cut back to doing the exercise only once.

Now write your own initial program and follow your progress using the exercise diary.

EXERCISE DIARY   Week of _____

Day	Figure Number	Number of Repetitions	Times a Day	Pain

6
Protecting Your Joints

Joint protection plays an important role in the management of arthritis, especially in rheumatoid arthritis. Because of inflammation or instability, arthritic joints may be unable to withstand the stresses applied during normal daily activities. Forces imposed from such simple activities as opening the car door, turning on the faucet, or climbing stairs may cause increased pain levels and may contribute to joint deterioration.

Joint protection is a means of using your joints wisely. In a broad sense, this entire book is about protecting your joints. Taking the appropriate medication, exercising your joints to their full range and strength, and eating a well-balanced diet are all ways of ensuring maximum joint function.

There are, however, some very specific principles that may be beneficial for your individual needs. These principles will help you to attain the three main goals of joint protection: (1) minimizing stress and pain, (2) maintaining mobility and function, and (3) conserving your energy.

MINIMIZING JOINT STRESS AND PAIN

What produces stress on a joint? Joint stress comes from factors such as time and force and depends on the type of arthritis. Strong forces over a short period of time or mild forces over long periods of time can contribute to further joint damage. For the arms and hands, a stressful force may occur during activities involving squeezing, pushing, pulling, twisting, and lifting movements. The weight-bearing joints—hips, knees, ankles, and feet—can be overstressed from either excessive body weight or activities that place increased loads on these joints. For example, walking on a level surface may not be bothersome, but getting up from a chair, climbing stairs, jogging, and carrying two grocery bags "load" these joints with more than body weight. The spine—back and neck—can be stressed by bending over, twisting while reaching for an object, and poor standing, sitting, or sleeping postures.

Overstressing a joint can contribute to intensified pain. In fact, the most common sign of joint stress is pain. Activity-induced pain is thus a warning sign for you to take it easier on that joint.

A painful joint is in many ways like a strained muscle. If in the initial stages of recovery the muscle is subjected to more activity than it can tolerate, the muscle will be more painful and will take longer to heal. On the other hand, a certain amount of movement by the muscle will facilitate the healing process. Optimum function for both the joint and the muscle is achieved by using the appropriate type and amount of activity. Both this joint protection and the exercise sections will assist you in determining the proper type and amount of activity for you.

Severe pain during a specific task or increased pain lasting for one to two hours after an activity should alert you to start the following steps:

1. Be aware of your body. Learn to recognize activity-induced pain.

2. Determine the particular movements that cause pain.

3. Use principles of joint protection to change the method of performing the activity.

The following principles are subdivided by the specific joints to which they apply. Select the principles that match your problem areas. Since learning new habits or new movement patterns takes time, begin by working with only one or two principles. As they are mastered, begin to incorporate additional principles into your daily routine.

PRINCIPLE 1   For Hands, Arms, and Back
Use the strongest or largest joint possible to accomplish a task.

This means that instead of using your fingers, use the palm of your hand, your forearm, or your elbow; instead of your arms, use your whole body; instead of your back, use your legs. In this way, the stress is distributed over the largest area possible. The larger the area, the more pressure, weight, and/or force the joint can tolerate.

Examples

Fingers

Spare your hands from difficult-to-open refrigerator doors or cupboards by placing a strap on the handle. To open, simply place your forearm through the strap and pull.

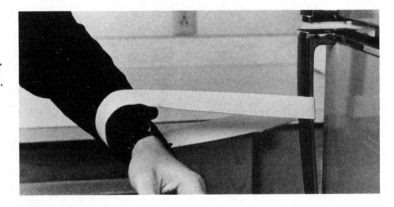

A doorknob extender allows you to open the door with the palm of the hand instead of with the fingers.

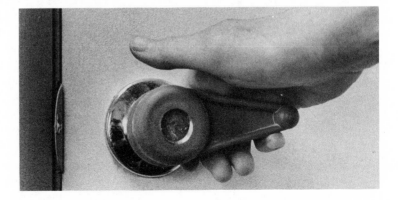

Hands and Elbows

Carry a purse on your forearm or use a shoulder bag to avoid clutching i
your hand.

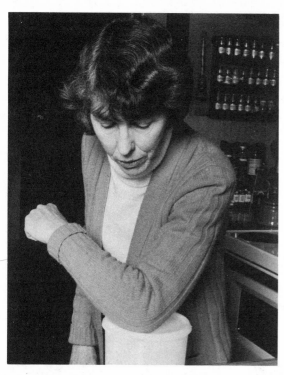

Close plastic containers with your elbow.

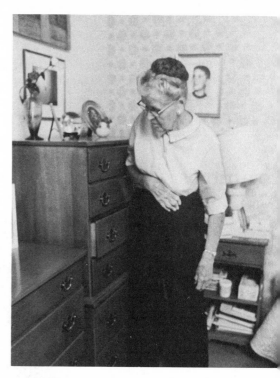

Use your hip to close kitchen or dresser
drawers.

Back

To lift heavy objects from the floor, bend your knees instead of the back.

PRINCIPLE 2   For the Hands, Arms, and Knees
Distribute the load over several joints.

This can often be accomplished by using both arms together to lift, push, o
pull objects. The concept is similar to principle 1, except that you want t
distribute the stress over as many joints as possible.

Examples
Hands and Arms

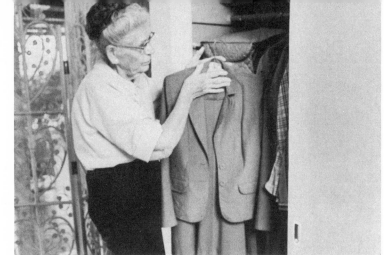

Use both arms to take down or hang clothes in the closet.

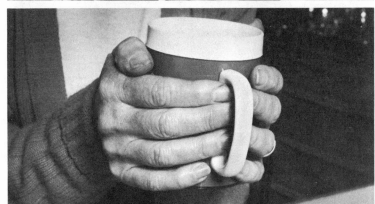

Instead of placing your fingers through the handle, encircle a coffee cup with both hands. Mugs are especially good for this.

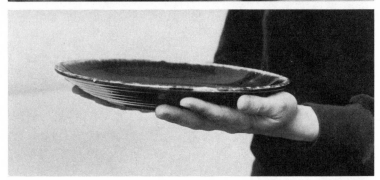

Carry your plate back to the kitchen by "scooping" it up with the palms of both hands.

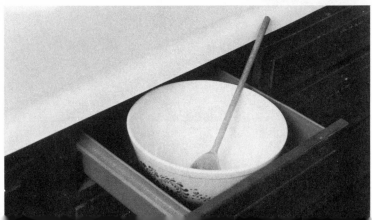

Use both hands to mix or stir by wedging the bowl in a drawer. Even better, of course, would be to use an electric mixer.

Examples

Knees

Sit in chairs with armrests so that you may push with your arms to stand up.

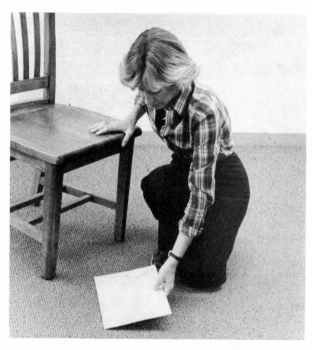

When stooping down to reach an object, use the edge of a chair or table to push up. (If your wrists or elbows are involved, however, you probably should avoid this because they may receive too much stress from your body weight.)

Use a luggage carrier when traveling. This allows you to take most of the strain off your arms as you push or pull the suitcase.

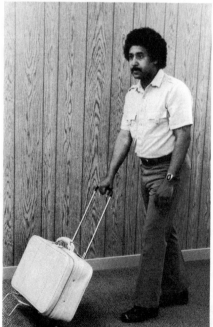

PRINCIPLE 3   For Hands, Arms, Knees, and Back

Use each joint in its most stable and functional position.

Each joint has a range in which it is most stable and from which it can work most effectively. This range is determined not only by the structure of the joint, but also by the muscles of the joint. Certain positions will allow for greater leverage and maximum efficiency of the muscles. These are usually positions where the joint is in a straight alignment, not bent or rotated to the side.

Examples

Knees

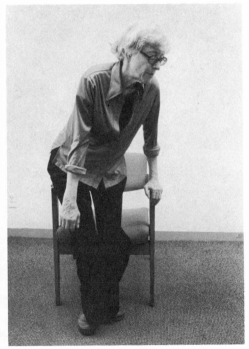
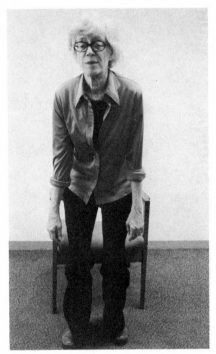

Wrong   **Right**

When standing up, keep both feet flat on the floor and pointed ahead. Stand straight up. Avoid pushing with one hand to prevent leaning to one side, causing harmful twisting strains on the knees.

Back

When opening a drawer, cupboard, or door, position yourself directly in front of it to prevent twisting of the trunk.

To pick up an object, make sure you face it directly, again to avoid twisting the trunk.

Hands

The position of your hand in relation to your forearm will determine the strength of your grip. Keep the hand in a straight alignment with the arm and bend the wrist backward slightly during most activities.

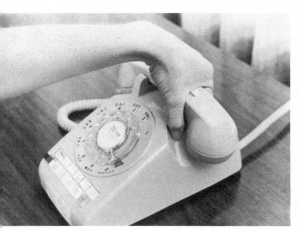

Wrong

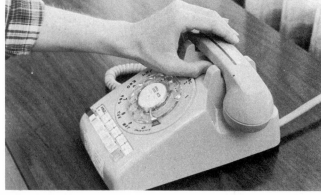

Right

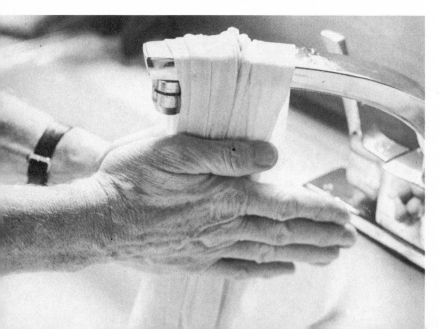

Wringing out wet washcloths or laundry places twisting motions on top of the strong pressures involved in squeezing. Wrap the item over the faucet and squeeze excess water out between the palms of your hands. An alternative is to wrap the item in a thick towel and let the towel soak up the excess moisture.

PRINCIPLE 4 Mostly for the Back and Neck
Use good body mechanics.

ody mechanics refers to the development of good posture and movement abits during daily activities. A key component of posture is the Pelvic Tilt, escribed earlier in the exercise section of Chapter 6 (exercise 28). The egree that the pelvis is tilted in relation to the spine helps determine how traight the spine is aligned. The better the alignment, the less strain on both nuscles and joints.

To feel this position, please refer to exercise 28 on page 46. While doing hese exercises, focus your awareness on the trunk and hips and try to maintain this position, the pelvic tilt, later during the day.

Examples

Standing

When standing for prolonged periods of time is necessary, alternate your ositions between the following:

Wrong   **Right**

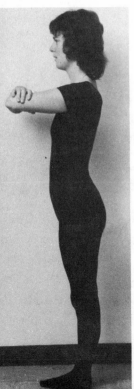 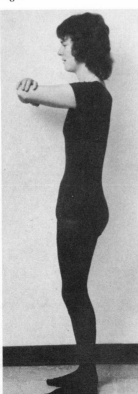

Stand with weight distributed equally between both feet. For a back problem, to assist with maintaining the pelvic tilt, avoid locking your knees. Don't do this if you also have a knee problem.

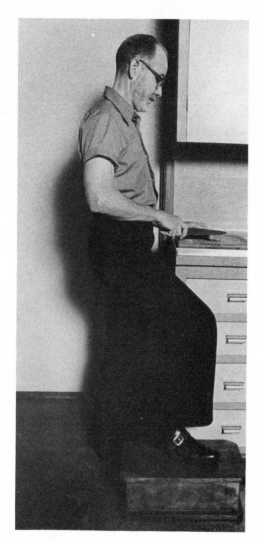

Place one foot on a footstool. This helps to maintain a pelvic tilt and thus alleviate low back strain.

Wear flat or low-heeled shoes, not only for the greater stability and safety they afford, but also because they help to keep the pelvis tilted.

Sitting

Select chairs that provide adequate support for your back. A firm seat and fairly straight back will help you to avoid slouching.

When writing at a desk, do not lean forward, but sit tall and bend the neck only slightly.

Persons with neck problems may want to consider a drafting table with an adjustable slant.

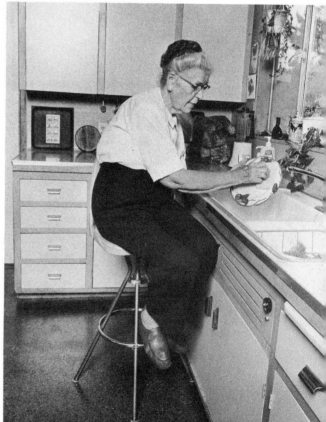

When working at your workbench or in the kitchen, a bar-height stool with footrest allows you to half-sit, half-stand. This helps to prevent fatigue, as well as to provide a suitable height for working on projects, washing dishes, or preparing meals.

Standing Up

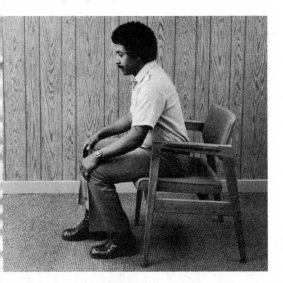

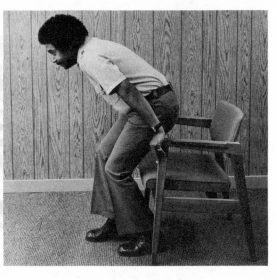

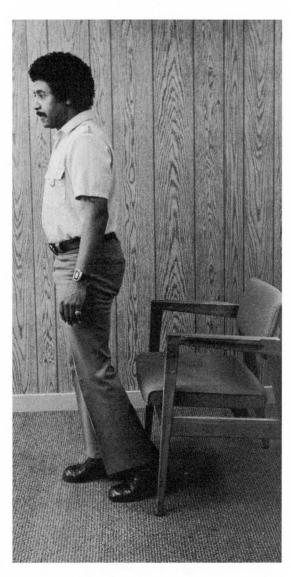

The most efficient method, utilizing good body mechanics and thus less muscle power, requires that you plan ahead. First, scoot forward in your chair so that you are near the edge. Second, place one foot slightly in front of the other so that it is directly under the knee. The other foot is behind the knee. Then lean forward until your hips automatically start to come off the chair.

Chairs that are several inches higher than normal, either through the use of pillows or chair leg extenders, make it easier to stand up.

Lifting

To lift objects from the ground or low shelves, bend your legs instead of your back; pick up the object, holding it as close to your body as possible, and rise, letting your leg muscles do the work.

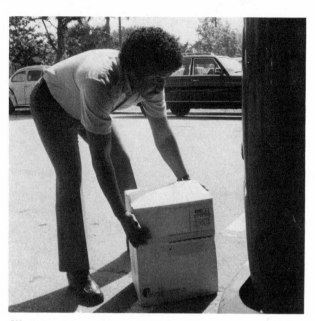

Wrong

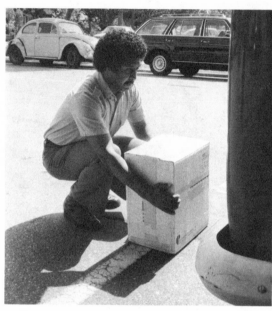

Right

Persons with knee involvement may want to let someone else lift heavy objects, since the knees will be strained from the weight of the object as well as from their own body weight.

PRINCIPLE 5
Reduce the effort required to do the job.

There are various ways to reduce the amount of effort we exert. In fact, all of the principles mentioned above involve this to some degree. However, there are some additional concepts that provide ways to modify either the tools or the activity itself.

These include: (1) using adaptive devices or tools suitable to the task, (2) employing leverage, and (3) avoiding lifting and carrying.

Examples

Use adaptive devices.

There are various aids or devices that have been developed for the express purpose of alleviating joint stress and pain. Others were developed to simplify all of our lives in one way or another, but they also act to protect joints. Some of these can be found in department or economy stores; others are available through either therapy departments or special catalogs. For information call or write the Arthritis Foundation in your area.

Examples of adaptive devices are illustrated at various points in this chapter, as well as in Chapter 7. The main point is that although it is not generally recommended that you accumulate a huge number of gadgets, it is important to make use of devices that will protect your joints. An occupational therapist can assist you in determining your equipment needs.

Employ leverage.

A piece of wood, metal, or firm plastic can be attached to many types of objects to increase the area for gripping. The longer the attachment or lever, the less pressure required to manipulate the desired object.

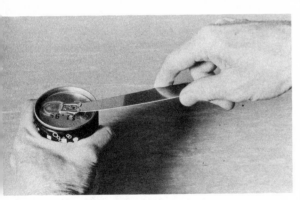

Open ring or flip-top cans with a knife.

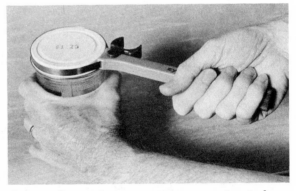

Certain types of jar openers are constructed with a long handle, thus employing the principle of leverage.

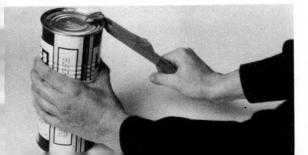

Attach a dowel or a piece of wood to a can opener and hold onto this lengthened handle when opening cans.

Avoid lifting and carrying.

Slide or push objects.

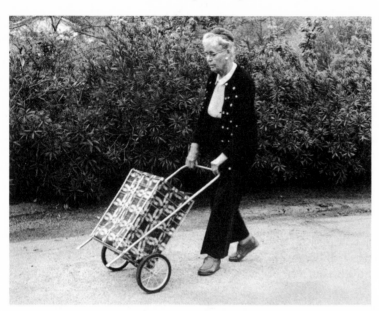

Use wheels to transport. Utility carts, tea tables, and shopping carts are just a few examples of readily available items on wheels.

"Deluxe" trash cans are now available that come equipped with wheels and a push handle. In addition, trash toters also have wheels in front and generally hold two regular-size trash cans.

MAINTAINING JOINT MOBILITY AND FUNCTION

The minimizing of joint stress and pain discussed above ties in directly with mobility and function. In the absence of pain, we are able to move our bodies freely—our bodies function well. When we experience pain, however, our natural reaction is to try to reduce it. Unfortunately, this is often accomplished by limiting movement and by keeping the affected joint in a bent position. This can produce a vicious cycle in which pain leads to an unwillingness to move, stiffness and shortening of muscles and joint tissues result, and there is a further increase in pain and difficulty with movement.

While minimizing pain is a crucial aspect of joint protection, one must be careful not to sacrifice mobility.

Wrong: disease ———→ dis-use ———→ dys-function

Right: dis-ease ———→ proper use ———→ maintain function

There are times, of course, when activities need to be limited. The rules for exercising a hot joint are applicable to activities. At these times, activities involving free and easy motions with little resistance are to be encouraged, while activities with resistance should be avoided. As the inflammation subsides, gradually work back to your normal level of activity.

PRINCIPLE 6   For Hips, Knees, Ankles, and Hands

Avoid prolonged periods of maintaining the same joint position.

There are two main points that illustrate the importance of this rule. First, joints affected by arthritis have a tendency to stiffen; this is sometimes referred to as the gel phenomenon. Therefore, frequent positions changes are essential to maintain mobility. Second, muscles that are fixed or tensed will fatigue. Fatigued muscles are not able to provide adequate support for your joints.

Examples

Hips and Knees

Alternate between sitting and standing positions. Although the sitting position is generally recommended to reduce stress on the lower joints and prevent fatigue, it is important to get up and stretch frequently.

Knees

When sitting, change the position of your legs so that your knees are often stretched out, feet supported by a footstool.

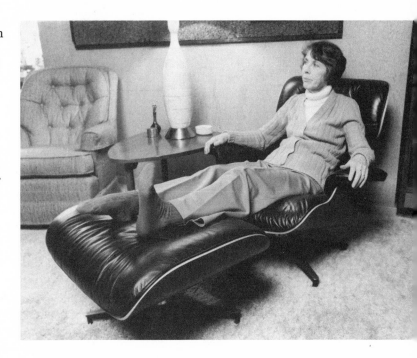

Ankles

Bend and point your toes while watching television or talking with a friend. You don't have to wait for a specific exercise time to do your range-of-motion exercises.

Hands

Avoid sustained grasps on objects. For example, instead of writing with a pen, use a typewriter.

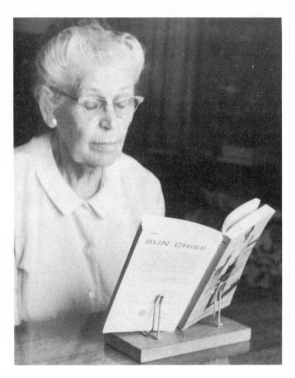 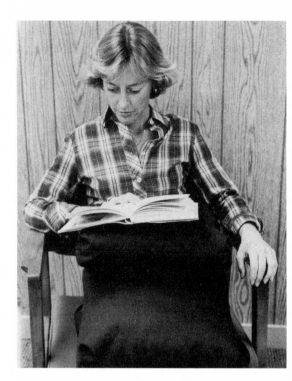

A book holder or pillows on your lap will serve as a means to support a book and will free your hands.

When it is necessary to maintain your grasp on an object for more than several minutes, take frequent breaks to stretch and move your fingers.

PRINCIPLE 7 For Arms

Encourage full and complete motions during daily activities.

Many daily activities, when performed correctly, provide movement patterns that can serve as an adjunct to your regular exercise program. They can stretch and strengthen. For example, long, sweeping, flowing strokes can help to maintain and increase the range of motion of a joint.

Examples
Shoulders

When ironing, straighten the arm as far as possible, using long, flowing strokes.

To vacuum, use a long, forward stroke with the vacuum, then pull it in close to the body so the arm is first fully straightened, then fully bent. If you have elbow or shoulder pain, however, you want to either walk with the vacuum cleaner as you move it forward or purchase the lightest model possible.

Encourage shoulder mobility by placing light objects on high shelves where you will have to reach to get them.

Reach as high as possible when washing windows.

PRINCIPLE 8   Primarily for the Knees, Arms, and Hands

Avoid positions and activities leading to possible joint deformities.

Deformities occur more frequently in rheumatoid arthritis than in any other kind of arthritis. Long-term disease may produce changes in joint structure, with consequent limitations of movement. When joint motion is limited, daily activities become difficult or, in some cases, impossible to perform.

As mentioned earlier, joints tend to be held in flexed or bent positions for comfort, which is a primary reason that deformities occur. Move out of such positions frequently. The following are examples of more appropriate postures.

Examples
Knees

Sleeping with pillows under the knees should be avoided unless otherwise advised.

When sitting, place your legs on a footrest to keep your knees straight for part of the time.

Elbows

Stretch your arms out in front of you or by your side when sitting or lying.

Hands

The hands, which contain intricate mechanisms, are prone to damage. The most common hand deformities of rheumatoid arthritis are swan's neck, ulnar deviation, and boutonniere.

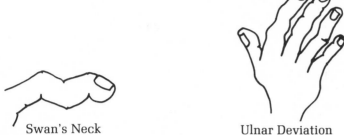

Swan's Neck   Ulnar Deviation   Boutonniere

There are several procedures to help prevent these deformities. These are reviewed below; however, consultation with an occupational therapist is recommended if you are beginning to develop these problems. The two subprinciples are:

PRINCIPLE 8A
Avoid excessive pressure against the back of the fingers, the pads of the thumb and fingers, and the thumb side of each finger.

Examples

The Back of the Fingers

When pushing up from a chair, keep your hands facing palm down.

Wrong   Right   Right

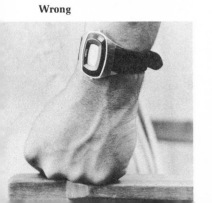
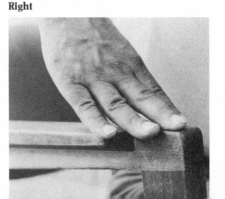
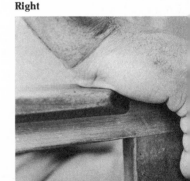

If you prop your chin in your hand, keep the palm of the hand toward your face.

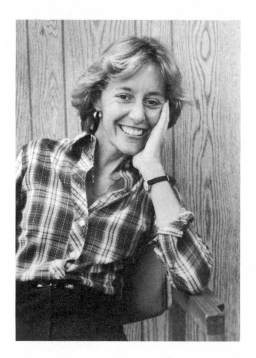

Right

The Pads of the Thumb and Fingers

When using spray cans or bottles, push down with the palm of the hand instead of the thumbtip.

Wrong

Right

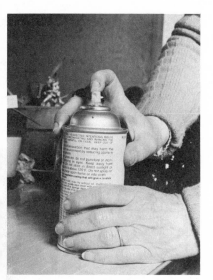

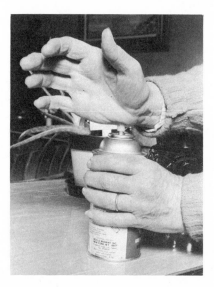

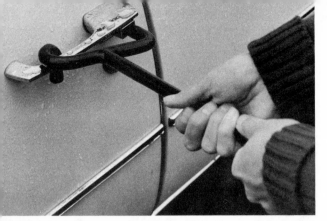

Open a car door with an aid in the palm of your hand.

Never use a butterfly can opener, because the pressure required to operate these is extreme; use an electric or wall-mounted type.

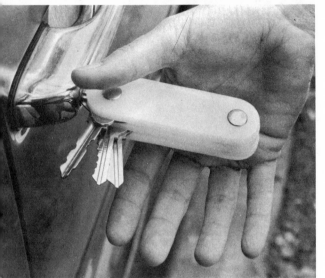

Special key holder devices allow you to turn a key by holding the handle in the palm of your hand. These are available through special-equipment firms or can be made by riveting a piece of wood or metal to the key.

The Thumb Side of Each Finger

To prevent ulnar deviation, turn jar lids, faucets, and doorknobs *toward* the thumb. This means that doors should be opened with the left hand and jars with the right.

Perform activities involving circular motions such as stirring, dusting, and washing dishes *toward* the thumb side of the hand. This is a counterclockwise motion with the right hand and clockwise with the left.

Use a wire-brush scourer with a handle to clean pots and pans. This allows you to hold the scourer in the palm of the hand instead of with the fingertips.

Try writing with the pencil held between the index and middle fingers.

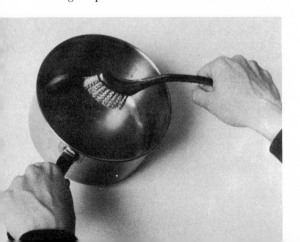

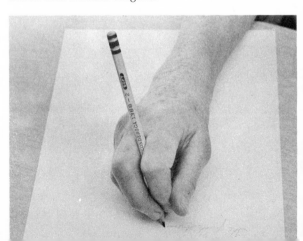

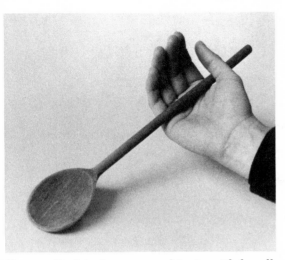
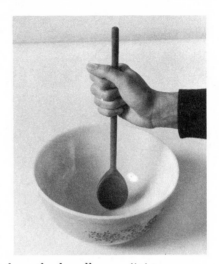

Use a cylindrical grasp on objects with handles; place the handle parallel to the knuckles. This includes such objects as mixing spoons, knives, tools, and brooms.

PRINCIPLE 8B
Avoid tight grasps on objects and keep hands open whenever possible.

Examples

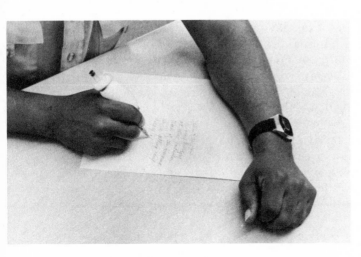

Foam padding added to such articles as a toothbrush, pen, razor, fork, and comb will increase the size of the handle. The larger the grip, the less tension required to maintain your hold on these objects.

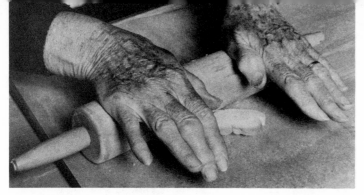

Instead of holding onto the handles of a rolling pin, place hands flat on top and roll beneath your hands.

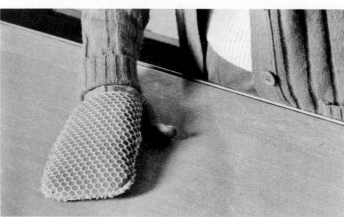

To wash dishes, there is a scrubber that fits over your hand available in supermarkets or hardware stores. Since you don't need to grasp it, you can keep your fingers in a straightened position.

Use a sponge instead of a dishrag to mop up tables and counters. The water can be squeezed out of the sponge more easily by putting it in the sink and pressing down with your flattened hand.

CONSERVING YOUR ENERGY

Did you conserve energy today? This question does not refer to natural resources such as gas and coal, but to your own body and its energy expenditures. A great deal of energy is expended unnecessarily by each of us in the normal course of the day. And just as natural resources are not easily replenished, neither are our own. If we work for several hours or a full day, we often don't have the energy in the evening to do more than collapse in front of the television. It would be nice to be able to pursue hobbies and other interests with as much energy as we felt earlier in the day.

Energy conservation techniques benefit all of us. Although much of it is simply common sense, energy conservation is actually a science that evolved from the desire to conserve energy and increase efficiency. Energy conservation techniques are particularly important for certain types of arthritis (notably rheumatoid), since feelings of fatigue and lethargy often accompany these diseases. In addition, energy conservation acts to protect joints by using your body efficiently, thus minimizing muscle fatigue, joint stress, and pain.

Several of the principles of energy conservation are briefly described below.

PRINCIPLE 9
Organize your work.

Each individual task, as well as each workday, can be organized ahead of time to prevent wasted time and motion. Try to get the most done with the least amount of effort.

Examples

"Think before you act." Develop your planning and organizing skills by starting with a pencil and paper and writing lists. Identify what needs to get done and in what order of importance. Focus on one or more particular tasks.

Combine several errands in one trip whenever possible. If you have to go upstairs or to another part of the house or place of work, try to accomplish several things at a time.

Plan for an easy flow of work by storing equipment and supplies where they will be used first; for example, keep pots for cooking vegetables near the sink or the stove.

Avoid rush by planning ahead. Hasty movements are often no more quickly accomplished than planned, purposeful movements, and they often end in extra work, as with the old adage, "Haste makes waste." Both tension and fatigue are increased when we feel rushed.

PRINCIPLE 10
Balance work with rest.

One of the most effective means of avoiding fatigue is to schedule short but frequent rest periods throughout the day. Resting before you get tired is often difficult because we all want to get our work done. If we can prevent fatigue, even if it means stopping in the middle of a job, our endurance over the long run will be increased. When stopping to rest is difficult to do, remember that long work periods require longer recovery periods.

Examples

Schedule frequent rest periods throughout the day. This will vary for each individual, but an example might be to rest ten minutes out of every hour, instead of working for three hours straight.

Alternate heavy and light work tasks during each day. In addition, plan the more difficult or lengthy tasks when you know you have the endurance to complete them.

Sitting to work is a form of rest since it uses less energy than standing
However, if you spend your workday behind a desk, you will find that moving
around at regular intervals will help to keep you more alert and energetic.

PRINCIPLE 11
Use efficient storage.

Efficient storage arrangements will help to (1) reduce the number of steps
you take to gather all the necessary supplies and (2) minimize bending,
stooping, and needless searching in unorganized places.

Examples

Determine easy-to-reach areas and use them for the most frequently used
supplies.

Store heavy items within easy reach, such as on countertops, and store
lighter items on the higher or lower shelves.

Organize storage areas with dividers, special racks, turntables, and pull-out
shelves. Many of these items are available in local stores or can be easily
made by a carpenter.

Use pegboards and hooks to hang objects.

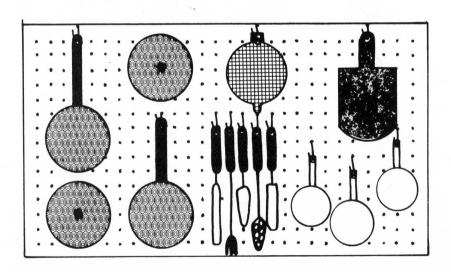

Have organized work centers for baking, clothes washing, hobbies, and so forth, where everything needed for a certain job is readily accessible. For example, a baking center can be set up with the flour, sugar, and other spices kept in the same cupborad with mixing bowls, measuring cups, and baking tins.

Remove unnecessary or infrequently used items from shelves.

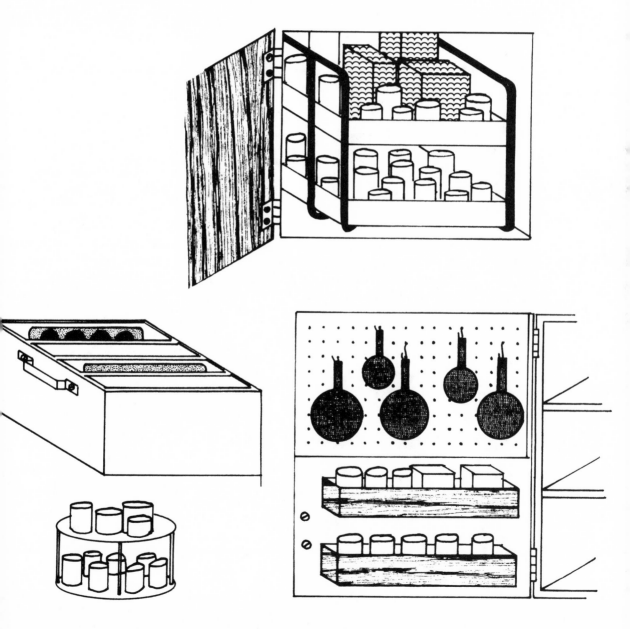

PRINCIPLE 12
Eliminate unnecessary tasks.

This is so self-explanatory it appears that no comments are necessary. "Voluntary simplicity" is a key to avoiding both stress and work.

Examples

If your homemaking standards for cleaning and cooking are higher than necessary, consider relaxing them to conserve energy.

Let dishes drip dry.

Use convenience foods or prepare foods in the easiest manner possible. For example, bake potatoes instead of mashing them.

Use the least amount of equipment possible. For example, measure the dry ingredients for a cake in a large two-cup measure and pour into the bowl. Next, measure and mix all the wet ingredients in the two-cup measure before adding to the dry ingredients. This eliminates an extra mixing bowl.

Realize that it is all right for you not to do everything and that you can ask family members to help you out. In fact, your family would probably prefer to lighten your load so that you can spend enjoyable, and not fatigued, time with them.

7
Self-Helpers
100 HINTS AND AIDS

The preceding chapter on joint protection provided you with basic principles and examples of how to protect your joints. Additional hints are provided in this chapter, not only on how to protect your joints, but also on how to do things if general mobility or finger coordination are impaired.

You may find that you already use many of the suggestions listed below. It is true that "necessity is the mother of invention." If you combine your needs and your common sense, you will probably come up with another 100 hints. Use these suggestions as a springboard for additional ideas to make your life easier and more comfortable. Then share them with friends and others who also could benefit from them.

DRESSING

If buttons are difficult to manipulate, sew Velcro on clothing, attach buttons permanently to the top side, and use the Velcro as a fastener. Velcro can be found in most sewing stores.

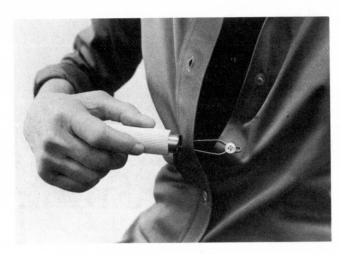

Buttonhooks work well to fasten buttons.

A final alternative for buttons on sleeves is to sew elasticized thread on button cuffs. This often provides sufficient give for your hands to slip through.

In the future, buy clothes that are easy to put on and easy to care for. Tops should be large enough or designed so that sleeves are easy to slip into—you may want to avoid turtlenecks. Elastic waistbands around pants should be loose enough to slip easily over hips. Fastenings should be located in the front and be easy to manipulate.

If reaching the clothes in the closet is difficult, have someone lower the rod.

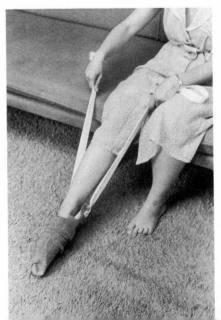

A stocking device will allow you to put socks on again if you can't reach your feet.

Special devices to assist with shoes include long-handled shoe horns, elastic shoelaces, and zipper laces.

A bent coat hanger, reacher, or dressing stick can assist with pulling pants up, straightening shirts, or retrieving clothes slightly out of reach.

Place large rings or leather loops on zipper tabs.

BATHING AND HYGIENE

A long-handled sponge or brush can be used to soap yourself when bathing.

Tub and shower benches, or an old kitchen chair, can allow you to sit while bathing. This helps to prevent fatigue and provides a place to sit when getting down into the tub is difficult.

Safety considerations when bathing include the use of nonskid safety strips or a rubber bathmat on the floor. In addition, grab bars can be permanently installed on the wall or attached to the edge of the bathtub. Grab bars assist with safety when climbing in and out of the tub or shower and also provide a place to pull or push up from when in the tub.

A long shower spray hose makes rinsing easier.

After bathing, put on a terry robe and let it soak up the water as you pat yourself dry.

Use a shower caddy to keep soap and shampoo within easy reach.

Bath mitts can be bought or easily made by sewing two facecloths together. Lather it up and soap yourself the easy way.

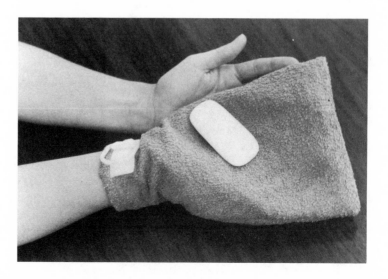

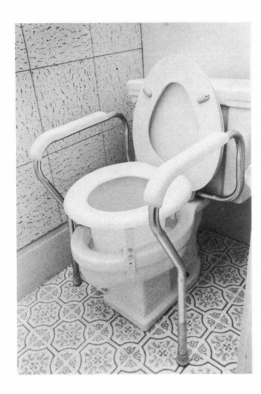

A raised toilet seat or commode over the toilet provides greater height and thus makes standing up easier.

In addition, a toilet safety frame or a grab bar installed in the wall next to the toilet will allow you to assist with your arms when sitting and standing.

Electric toothbrushes and Water-Piks make oral hygiene easier. In addition, there is a device that holds dental floss, allowing you to floss your teeth with one hand holding onto the handle—ask your dentist about this or check you local drugstore.

Special long-handled combs and brushes are useful when shoulder and elbow limitations prevent reaching your head.

COOKING

Microwave ovens save time and energy. They are easy to operate, easy to clean, and easy to reach since they are usually placed on countertops. In addition, you do not need to worry about burning yourself since only the food heats up.

To avoid lifting pots heavy with food and the water it was boiled in, there are several alternatives. One is to place a frying basket inside a pot so that you may lift the food out with the basket and drain the water later. Spaghetti cookers come with a perforated insert and can serve in the same manner. Or you may want to ladle the contents out.

To open jars, install a jar opener that will grip the lid as you use both hands to turn the jar itself. Also, ask other members of the family not to close lids too tightly.

Use lightweight cooking utensils, bowls, and dishes. Avoid cast iron skillets and heavy ceramic bowls.

Select appliances with levers or push buttons that are easy to operate.

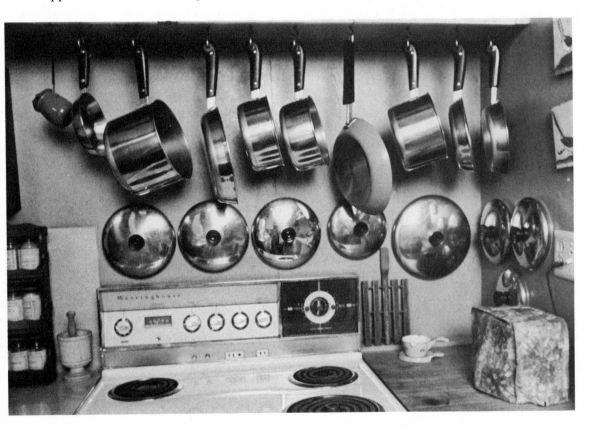

Use efficient storage arrangements. Have a "French kitchen" with pots, pans, and frequently used utensils hanging from the ceiling or wall fixtures.

Plan and prepare meals ahead of time to avoid last-minute preparations. Cook some meals the day before, let the flavors enhance, and then heat them up again the next day. Also, try preparing double or triple portions and freeze the extra.

Use cookie tins and pans with special surfaces that prevent sticking and messy cleanup, or spray them with a nonstick product.

Mixing bowls can be stabilized by placing on a wet washcloth or on little octopus suction cups.

Place flour and sugar in containers so you can scoop out the amount needed and avoid lifting heavy bags each time.

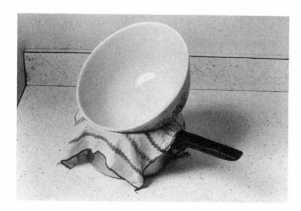

Use a pot with a wet cloth draped over it as a support for a bowl when pouring batter into a baking pan.

Mitt pot holders allow you to lift hot pans with the palms of both hands.

Use a bent coat hanger or dowel with a hook to pull oven shelves out when checking on the meal.

Attach a spray hose at the kitchen sink so that you can fill pots with water on the countertop; slide pots to the stove to avoid lifting.

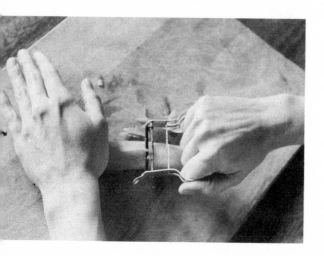

When peeling vegetables, try the kind of peeler with a handle you can slip your fingers through.

Instead of slicing onions, use an onion chopper.

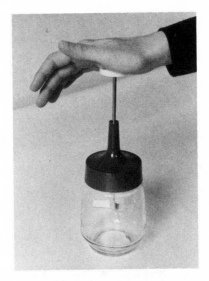

Try using a pizza wheel to cut various foods.

Food processors, the latest item to revolutionize the art of cooking, make food preparation a snap, especially when large quantities of food must be chopped, sliced, or grated.

HOUSEKEEPING

Keep a set of cleaning supplies in each area where they are used to eliminate needless walking.

To clean the bathtub, sit on a low stool next to the tub and use a long-handled sponge.

Long-handled sponges can also be used to clean around door sills and other hard-to-reach places.

Use a long-handled dustpan and small broom to clean up dry spills from floors.

Use an adjustable-height ironing board so that you can sit to iron. Attach a cord-minder to keep the cord out of your way.

Carpeting or foam-backed rugs help to ease ankle and foot pain when prolonged standing and moving about are necessary.

Use gravity whenever possible. Let your clothes fall from the dryer into the basket. When scooping them out, you may want to use a reacher or stick.

Laundry bags that were originally intended for washing delicate items like nylons can be used for all small pieces of clothing (socks, underwear) and thus eliminate searching in the machine.

If lifting detergent boxes is difficult, you can either have someone else pour some into a smaller container or buy the 20-pound size and scoop it out. Liquid detergents may also be more manageable.

Try using the old-style push-on clothespins rather than pinch clothespins.

Front-loading washers are generally easier to use than top-loading washers. Raising the washer on blocks will also make laundering easier, since bending is eliminated.

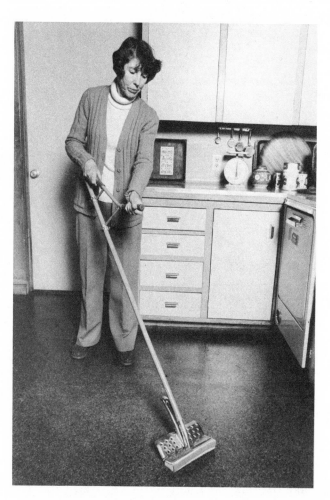

Use a Back Preserver tool on your floor mop or push broom. These tasks can be performed with better posture and less strain to the back with this special long-handled attachment.

If fitted sheets are difficult to manage, slit the last corner and fasten with a tie.

Use an oven shovel to tuck in sheets.

DRIVING

Auxiliary or wide-angle mirrors allow for increased visibility when neck movement is limited.

Special spinner knobs can be attached to the steering wheel to make steering easier when holding the wheel in the normal position is difficult.

To make driving more comfortable and to prevent low back strain, you may want to look into Sacro Ease seats, which are especially suitable for cars. They are similar to the cooling cushion inserts used when driving during the summer, but can be bent to fit your body curvatures and support your low back.

RECREATION OR LEISURE TIME

The best form of physical activity is swimming, since the buoyancy of the water helps to support the joints. In addition, much of your normal exercise routine can be performed while in the water. Check with the pools in your area to see if any of them provide "therapeutic pool" times, with water temperatures between 87 and 92 degrees.

An embroidery frame that can be attached to a table or chair will allow you to do needlework and sewing without using your hands to stabilize the article. These are available primarily through self-help aids catalogs.

If you like to play cards, try using a card holder. These can be purchased through mail-order catalogs or easily made by sawing a slit in a piece of wood.

If you enjoy gardening, there is now an attachment for shovels. There is a different attachment to be used with hoes and rakes. These Back Preserver tools can easily be attached to your own equipment.

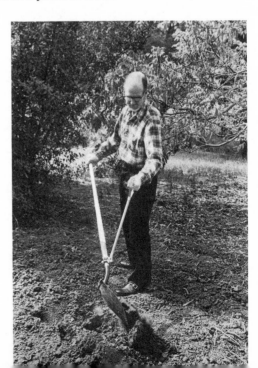

When gardening, try sitting on a small stool instead of kneeling to weed and plant.

Gardening can be made even easier by having a planter box or raised flower beds made. This will eliminate stooping entirely, as you can sit to work at a comfortable level.

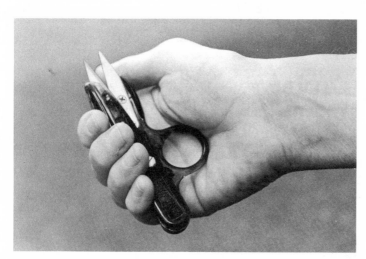

Use special clipping scissors when sewing to avoid pressure and pain on the thumb joint.

If threading a needle is difficult, self-threading needles or automatic threading machines are available through catalogs and in some sewing stores.

Afternoon exercises or sports are a really good way to break up the day. Try to set up a schedule at work where you can take an extended break to swim or exercise during the lunch hour.

JOINT WARM-UP (TO KEEP JOINTS WARM)

Use the extra-long heating pads that wrap around an arm or leg and fasten with Velcro to warm an elbow or knee.

Soak stiff, sore, or cold hands in warm water. This is especially useful to loosen them from morning stiffness. At night, warm the hands in this manner; rub hand lotion in and wear cotton gloves while sleeping.

Thermoelastic gloves are especially warming, since they are made from wool and elastic fibers. They are available in some pharmacies.

Thermoelastic products are also available for knees and elbows. A soft, thick knee sock could also be used in the same manner. Cut the sock so you have a tube approximately seven inches long and place the tube over your knee or elbow.

Use electric blankets as a lightweight cover; they are especially useful in warming the bed before you get in it.

An alternative way to stay warm during the night or when resting is to sleep inside a sleeping bag that is placed under a blanket. The bag will turn with you and prevent cold air spaces.

Use a sleeping bag, cozy-wrap, or comforter when reading in a chair.

Use a mug to drink hot tea or coffee and hold it between both hands to warm them.

Slipper socks, worn over a pair of regular socks, will help to keep feet and ankles warm.

A new product on the market is the foot bath, which not only will warm your feet as they soak in the water but also can act as a massager.

Dress warmly. Use long underwear even in the spring and fall.

Place a space heater or heat lamp in your bathroom and turn it on before showering in the morning.

Stand by the radiator to warm up, or build a fire in the fireplace.

COMFORT

When sitting for long periods of time is necessary, such as when flying, you can relax your back muscles by doing the following. Place your forearms on your thighs, hands near the knees, and lean forward with your face as near to the knees as possible. Breathe deeply and relax in this position. Repeat several times.

Purchase a padded toilet seat, or sew a cover for it out of thick, furry material.

Pad chairs with pillows or foam cushions.

If you don't want to take a pillow with you when going out, take a sweater or jacket along to use as a cushion for hard chairs.

Pain at the base of the toes may be alleviated by placing a bar behind the ball of the foot on the shoe sole. This will allow you to avoid the painful area by rolling off the bar. You should talk to your doctor, podiatrist, or physical therapist about this before experimenting. It is called a *metatarsal bar*.

Painful feet may also benefit from orthopedic inserts. Ask your physician or podiatrist about them.

Recliner chairs with head supports are comfortable for many people, especially if you have neck problems.

Electric beds are no longer confined to the hospital. Home models are available that have movable back and foot sections.

Be sure that you have adequate lighting and ventilation for all activities.

If you take aspirin for pain, you may want to wake up earlier than necessary, take your aspirin, and go back to sleep until it begins to work. Keep aspirin and a glass of water at the bedside.

Splints, often made for hands and from special plastics, help to maintain proper joint alignment, prevent stress, and reduce pain. Your physician can refer you to an occupational therapist who can construct one for you.

An Ace bandage can also provide some added stability to joints, as well as serve as a reminder to protect them.

MISCELLANEOUS

To control lamps, equipment, and appliances in inaccessible locations, there is a plug on the market with an on-off switch. This can plug in directly to a wall outlet or can be attached to an extension cord that can be positioned near you.

An easier, though quite expensive, method of controlling appliances and lights is with a Home Control Unit. Available through certain large department stores, this device consists of a command console and up to 16 module units for each appliance wanted. Pushing the buttons on the console will turn any appliance on or off anywhere in your house.

Use a clipboard to keep writing paper steady.

A felt-tip pen allows you to write with less pressure.

Reachers extend your reach from two to three feet, allowing you to retrieve from the floor or on high shelves.

When attending lectures, use a cassette recorder to eliminate note taking.

When shaking hands with another person, grasp the fingers of the person's hands first so that his or her thumb cannot grasp and squeeze your hand too hard.

Use a steak or paring knife at dinner since the sharper the knife, the less pressure needed. Be careful.

Make sure that the chairs you use at home are easy to get out of—if not, you may not want to get out of them often enough to move around and loosen up. Avoid soft, low chairs.

Dialing a phone may be easier with a pencil held in the palm of the hand. Also, check with the phone company, which now has interesting and easy-to-operate models.

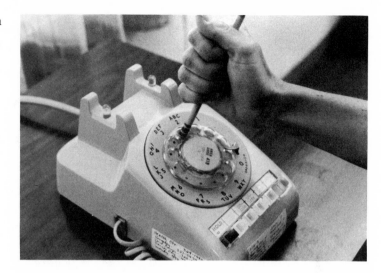

Enlarged knobs are available to place on lamps as well as appliances such as washing machines (certain brands only) to increase ease of handling. Check with your washing-machine manufacturer if the controls are difficult to operate.

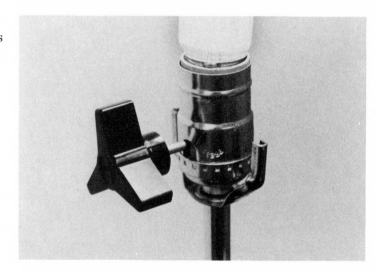

8
Relaxation Techniques

So much has been said and written about relaxation that most of us are completely confused. It is not a cure-all, but neither is it a hoax. Rather, like most treatment methods, it has specific uses in the management of arthritis. The advantage of relaxation is that your muscles become less tense and thus it is easier and less painful to move the joints. In addition to the release of residual tension throughout the body, these techniques are useful in helping you sleep. Relaxation exercises seem to be particularly helpful in relieving pain.

Like exercise, the following techniques take practice. Thus, if you do not feel you are accomplishing anything, be patient and keep trying. Feel free to try another method if the one you have chosen does not seem to work for you, but give it a full week trial. Relaxation techniques can be practiced at any time of the day. With many forms of arthritis, it is wise to take short rest periods during the day to avoid undue fatigue and to relieve stress on the joints. This is an excellent time to practice relaxation techniques.

The following are examples of relaxation techniques. Once you choose the one that works best for you, it may be helpful to tape record the technique. This is not necessary but is sometimes helpful if you find it hard to concentrate or follow the routine. With an inexpensive cassette recorder you can make a tape to follow so that you don't have to think hard or look at this book while you are trying to relax.

JACOBSON PROGRESSIVE RELAXATION

Many years ago, a psychiatrist, Edmund Jacobson, discovered that if a person wants to relax he or she must learn what it feels like to be relaxed and to be tense. Thus, he designed a very simple set of exercises to assist with the learning process. Jacobson felt that if one could recognize tension he or she could then let it go and relax. Progressive relaxation is best done lying on your back either on a rug or in bed. However, it can be done seated in a comfortable chair. Choose a quiet time and place where you will not be disturbed for at least fifteen minutes.

Technique for Progressive Relaxation of Each Muscle Group

First, for each muscle group of the arms and shoulders:

- Tense (contract) the muscles, holding until the tension is located (two to five seconds).

- Feel the tension, notice it carefully.

  Now release, let the tension slide away, all away.

- Feel the difference.

- Notice the pleasant warmth of relaxation.

- Repeat this sequence with the same group, but use only about half the tension.

- Repeat again with the same muscle group, but allow little movement so that only slight tension can be detected.

For the muscle groups of the lower limbs, trunk, and face it is only necessary to tense the muscles once, very slightly—just enough to recognize the tension. Then let it slide away. Feel the difference. Notice the pleasant warmth of relaxation.

MUSCLE GROUPS	TENSION EXERCISES
1. Dominant hand	Lift hand and make a fist; relax.
Other hand	Lift hand and make a fist; relax.

2. Dominant arm	Lift arm at shoulder; relax.
Other arm	Lift arm at shoulder; relax.
3. Shoulders	Shrug shoulders; relax.

Repeat each of the above three times with progressively less tension.

4. Right foot	Bend toes, relax; lift toes, relax.
Left foot	Bend toes, relax; lift toes, relax.
5. Right leg	Start to bend knee (drag heel up slightly); relax.
Left leg	Start to bend knee (drag heel up slightly); relax.
6. Buttocks	Squeeze together; relax.
7. Abdomen	Make abdomen tight and hard; relax.
8. Chest and neck	Squeeze shoulder blades together and slightly arch back, pressing head backward; relax.
9. Breathing	Take a slow deep breath and relax completely as you exhale. Repeat two or three times.
10. Upper face and scalp	Raise eyebrows; relax. Close eyes tightly; relax.
11. Center face	Scowl and wrinkle nose; relax. Widen cheeks and brow; relax.
12. Lower face	Purse lips; relax. Smile; relax. Drop jaw; relax.
13. Breathing	Take a slow deep breath and relax completely as you exhale. Repeat two or three times.

Technique for Progressive Relaxation of the Whole Body*

■ Tense all the muscles together and hold for five seconds.

■ Feel the tension, notice it carefully, then release. Let all the tension slide away.

---

* Much of this section has been adapted from Gordon Paul, *Insight vs. Desensitization, An Experiment in Anxiety Reduction* (Stanford, Calif.: Stanford University Press, 1966).

- Notice any remaining tension. Release it.

- Take a deep breath. Say "relax" softly to yourself as you breathe out slowly.

- Remain totally relaxed.

- Repeat breathing in and out slowly, saying "relax," staying perfectly relaxed.

- Do this three times.

- The exercise has ended—enjoy the relaxation.

Jacobson emphasizes that the only purpose of voluntarily tensing the muscles is to learn to recognize and locate the tension in your body. Hopefully, you will then become aware of the minor states of involuntary tension and use the same procedure of letting go. Once learned it is unnecessary to tense voluntarily, just locate the tension and let it go.

For people with very painful joints, the Jacobson technique may not be the best exercise for relaxation. If it causes any pain, the pain may distract from the relaxation. If this is the case for you, try the following techniques

THE RELAXATION RESPONSE

During the early 1970s, Dr. Herbert Benson did extensive work on what he calls the relaxation response. He says that our bodies have several natural states. For example, if you meet a lion on the street, you will probably become quite tense. In fact, the response will be a "fight or flight" response. After extreme tension, the body's natural response is to relax. This is what happens after a sexual climax. As life has become more and more complex, our bodies tend to stay in a constant state of tension. Thus, to elicit the relaxation response, many people need to consciously practice the following exercise.

Four Basic Elements

1. **A quiet environment.** "Turn off" not only internal stimuli but also distractions.

2. **An object to dwell upon or a mental device,** for example, repeating a word or sound like the word *one*, gazing at a symbol like a flower, or concentrating on a feeling, such as peace.

3. **A passive attitude.** This is the most essential factor. It is an emptying of all thoughts and distractions from your mind. Thoughts, imagery, and

feeling may drift into awareness—don't concentrate on them, but allow them to pass on.

4. **A comfortable position.** You should be comfortable enough to remain in the same position for 20 minutes.

Technique for Eliciting the Relaxation Response

1. Sit quietly in a comfortable position.

2. Close your eyes.

3. Deeply relax all your muscles, beginning at your feet and progressing up to your face. Keep them relaxed.

4. Breathe in through your nose. Become aware of your breathing. As you breathe out through your mouth, say the word *one* silently to yourself. Try to empty all thoughts from your mind, concentrate on *one*.

5. Continue for 10 to 20 minutes—you may open your eyes to check the time, but do not use an alarm. When you finish, sit quietly for several minutes, at first with your eyes closed. Do not stand up for a few minutes.

6. Do not worry about whether you are successful in achieving a deep level of relaxation. Maintain a passive attitude and permit relaxation to occur at its own pace. When distracting thoughts occur, try to ignore them by not dwelling upon them, and return to repeating *one*.

7. Practice once or twice daily, but ideally not within two hours after any meal, since digestive processes seem to interfere with elicitation of relaxation responses.

You may have noticed that this exercise is very much like meditation. In fact, meditation has provided the principles of the relaxation response. There is no need to spend several hundred dollars to learn to meditate. You now know all the steps.

SELF-MASSAGE

Self-massage can be considered a relaxation technique and an aid in managing arthritis. Its benefits include the release of tension, the preparation of the body for exercise by relaxing muscles and joints, and the increase of the circulation of blood throughout the body. Furthermore, proper self-massaging can provide comforting heat and warmth to an affected joint.

Self-massage is a simple procedure and can be performed well with little preparation or practice. For instance, no equipment is necessary; a comfortable position is all you need, so as to reach the desired area of massage. Therefore, you can do self-massage at home, at your place of work, or even while waiting at a stoplight. Massage or baby oil can help your hands to move smoothly over the skin, but oil is not at all necessary. Also, self-massage can be done effectively without even removing your clothes.

The techniques of self-massage include: (1) kneading, as if you were preparing dough to bake in the oven; (2) deep pressure in firm circular motions; and (3) firm pressure with fingertips pressing deeply into the muscles. You can combine these techniques to gain the desired relaxation in your joints.

Now, all you need to do is explore and experiment to find the area of tension and the proper technique for release and relaxation. Try self-massage on your neck, back, shoulders, legs, feet, and fingers.

For information on techniques for specific areas or for massage with a partner, you may want to refer to *The Massage Book,* by George Downing (New York: Random House, 1972).

These and other varieties of relaxation (such as hypnosis, self-hypnosis, biofeedback, and autogenic training) are not "scientifically proven" treatments for arthritis, and we make no special claims for them. Many individuals in our classes report substantial benefit from these practices, however, and we feel that they have merit for some if used as an adjunct to and not a substitute for a basic sound program.

A word of caution: Various relaxation techniques are often sold in expensive packages as a cure-all for almost everything. Such expensive courses are not necessary. If you want to take a relaxation course, check the following points to avoid unnecessary expense and disappointment.

1. Is the course offered by a reputable institution?

2. Is the cost reasonable? (Five to seven dollars an hour for small group instruction is about average.)

3. Are claims or promises made for a cure? If so, look elsewhere.

9
Getting a Good Night's Sleep

Sleep is vital for a healthy outlook toward life and important in caring for ourselves. A comfortable bed that allows ease of movement is the first requirement for a good night's sleep. This usually means a firm mattress of good quality that does not allow the body to sag in the middle of the bed. A bedboard, made of 3/8-1/2 inch plywood, can be placed between the mattress and the box spring to increase firmness. Bedboards can be bought commercially or constructed at home.

A heated waterbed is helpful for some people with arthritis because it supports weight evenly by conforming to the body's shape and because it distributes heat to the joints and muscles. Others find waterbeds uncomfortable, even to the point of generating seasickness. If you are interested, try one out at a friend's home or a hotel for a few nights to decide if it is right for you.

An electric blanket, used at a low heat, is another effective way of providing heat while sleeping, especially for cool or damp nights. If you decide to use one, be sure to read and follow the instructions carefully.

Pillows can be used to increase comfort and provide support. For maximum neck comfort, a small pillow should support the curvature of the neck. A pillow can be placed under the shoulder or, if you are lying on your side, under the upper arm to reduce stress on the shoulder joint. For low back problems, a pillow can be placed under the knees, though this position should not be used continuously for a lengthy period of time. Do not place a pillow under your knees or ankles if you have a knee or hip problem.

Positions that are not recommended if you have a disc problem are lying flat on your back or sleeping face down. A recommended position is the side-lying position, in which you lie on your side with knees bent. In this position it can be helpful to place a pillow between the knees to alleviate stress on the hips and low back. A pillow can also be placed under the upper arm to reduce stress on the shoulder joint. But in most cases your body will tell you the best position. There is no single right way.

If you have ankylosing spondylitis, there are some specific sleep positions that will help prevent deformity and loss of mobility of the spine. Sleep on your stomach or flat on your back. Avoid using high pillows under your head; sleep without a pillow if possible. Place a small pillow between your shoulder blades when you sleep on your back.

Sedatives and sleeping pills should be used with great caution. They are often habit forming, they suppress important stages of sleep, and they may cause depression. They only rarely solve sleep problems; the medication that is taken to control sleep actually may produce a disturbed night's sleep. When you stop them, do so gradually. This is also true of alcohol, which some people use as a sleeping medication.

Anti-inflammatory drugs should be taken as prescribed, with the proper dose taken at bedtime. Painkillers are less desirable and should be used with caution because they do not cure the arthritis but only temporarily suppress the symptoms.

Insomnia is a problem that affects all of us at one time or another. However, it can be a cause of concern if it occurs frequently and involves recurrent daytime fatigue or depression. The causes of insomnia are many, some of which are feelings of anxiety or worry, pain or discomfort due to a medical condition, or an unfamiliar sleeping environment. Other contributing factors may be improper self-treatment or failure to follow the practitioner's recommended dosage or directions for medications. If your sleeping problem continues, you may want to seek a physician's advice. One note: Older persons need less sleep, so be sure your insomnia is not due to sleeping too much. There is more worry about sleeping problems than there are problems.

Some hints for a more comfortable night's sleep include:

- Maintain a regular sleep schedule so that you go to bed and awaken at about the same time each night and morning.

■ Use some of the relaxation techniques described in this book or create one of your own that is particularly relaxing to you and will settle the day's thoughts and ease the body's tensions.

■ Wait until you are sleepy and your body is ready and eager to go to sleep; going to bed early to ensure a good night's sleep is often counter-productive.

■ Avoid caffeine (coffee, tea, soft drinks, chocolate) for several hours before bedtime because it can act as a stimulant.

■ Moderate your alcohol intake; alcohol may cause an erratic night's sleep and restlessness.

■ Provide yourself with a comfortable environment. Your environment includes mattress, lighting, noise level, temperature, and ventilation.

■ Try taking a warm bath before going to bed.

If you do wake up with stiffness, try some of the easier exercises of Chapter 5 (or small movements in the pain-free range) right in the bed to reduce discomfort and pain, allowing for a more undisturbed and restful sleep.

For more information on restful sleep, refer to *Insomnia: The Guide for Troubled Sleep*, by Gay Gaer Luce and Julius Segal (Garden City, N.Y.: Doubleday, 1969), or *How to Get a Good Night's Sleep*, by Richard Turbo (Boston: Little, Brown, 1978).

10
Depression and Other Problems

Depression is like waking up under a big dark cloud every day. Just when you think that you have it licked, back comes the depression, greater than ever.

One of the most frequent problems associated with arthritis is depression. Depression and pain and concerns about growing old are often part of a vicious cycle. The more depressed you are, the more pain you feel; the more pain you feel, the more depressed you become.

We have already discussed a number of ways to deal with pain, including heat, relaxation, exercise, and medications. It is when you are the most depressed that you need to pay the most attention to these techniques. Continue to do these things when you are feeling well in order to maintain your good spirits. Take your medicine and do your exercises—even if you don't feel like it. But you also want to lick the depression that is making everything worse.

It is not hard to tell when you have pain. But it is not as easy to recognize when you are depressed. Just as there are many degrees of pain, so there are many different degrees of depression. If your arthritis is a significant problem, you almost certainly have or have had some problems with depression; such problems are normal. Depression is felt by everyone at some time. It is how you handle it that makes the difference. The following 14 signs have to do with depression, and you probably have had some of them, in either mild or severe form. Learn them, because they are not the disease but the reaction to the disease, and you need to be able to cope with them.

1. Loss of interest in friends of activities. Not "being home" to friends, perhaps not even answering the doorbell.

2. Isolation. Not wanting to talk to anyone, only watching television, avoiding friends that you happen to meet on the street.

3. Difficulty sleeping, changed sleeping patterns, interrupted sleep, or sleeping more than usual. Often, going to sleep easily, but awakening and being unable to return to sleep. (It is important to remember that older people need less sleep.)

4. Loss of interest in food.

5. Loss of interest in personal care and grooming.

6. Unintentional weight change, either gain or loss, or more than ten pounds in a short period of time.

7. A general feeling of unhappiness lasting longer than six weeks.

8. Loss of interest in being held or in more intimate sex. These problems can sometimes be due to medications and they are very important, so be sure to talk them over with your doctor.

9. Suicidal thoughts. If your unhappiness has caused you to think seriously about killing yourself, get some help from your doctor, good friends, a minister or priest, a psychologist, or a social worker. These are not things to kill yourself over, and these feelings will pass and you will feel better. So get help and don't let a tragedy happen.

10. Frequent accidents. Watch for a pattern of increased carelessness, accidents while walking or driving, dropping things, and so forth.

11. Low self-image. A feeling of worthlessness, a negative image of your body, wondering if it is all worth it. This too will pass.

12. Frequent arguments. A tendency to blow up easily over minor matters, over things that never bothered you before.

13. Loss of energy. Feeling tired all of the time.

14. Inability to make decisions. Feeling confused and unable to concentrate.

If some of these seem familiar, you may well be depressed. There are at least 11 things that you can do to change the situation. But, being depressed, you may not feel like making the effort. Force yourself or get someone to help you into action. Find someone to talk with. Here are the 11 actions:

1. If you feel like hurting yourself or someone else call your mental health center, doctor, suicide prevention center, a friend, clergyman, or senior center. Do not delay. Do it now. These feelings do not mean that you are crazy. Most of us feel this way at one time or another. Often, just talking with an understanding person or health professional will be enough to help you through this mood.

2. Are you taking tranquilizers? These include drugs such as Valium, Librium, reserpine, codeine, sleeping medications, and other "downers." These drugs intensify depression, and the sooner you can stop taking them, the better you will be. Your depression may well be a drug side effect. If you are not sure what you are taking or what the side effects might be, check with your doctor or pharmacist. Before discontinuing a prescription medication, always check, at least by phone, with the prescribing physician, as there may be important reasons for continuing its use or there may be withdrawal reactions.

3. Are you drinking alcohol in order to feel better? Alcohol is also a downer. There is virtually no way to escape depression unless you unload your brain from these negative influences. For most people, one or two drinks in the evening is not a problem, but if your mind is not totally free of alcohol during most of the day you are having trouble from this drug.

4. Continue your daily activities. Get dressed every day, make your bed, get out of the house, go shopping, walk your dog. Plan and cook meals. Force yourself to do these things even if you don't feel like it.

5. Visit with friends. Call them on the phone, plan to go to the movies or on other outings. Do it.

6. Join a group. Get involved in a church group, a discussion group at a YWCA or YMCA, a senior citizen club, a community college class, a self-help class, or a senior nutrition program.

7. Make plans and carry them out. Look to the future. Plant some young trees. Look forward to your grandchildren's graduation from college even if they are in kindergarten.

8. Don't move to a new setting without first visiting for a few weeks. Moving can be a sign of withdrawal, and depression often intensifies when you are in a location away from friends and acquaintances. Your troubles may move, too.

9. Take a vacation with relatives or friends. Vacations can be as simple as a few days in a nearby city or a resort just a few miles down the road. Rather than go alone, look into trips sponsored by colleges, the American Association of Retired People, or church groups.

10. Do 10 to 15 minutes of physical exercise every day.

11. Make a list of self-rewards. Take care of yourself. You can reward yourself by reading at a set time, seeing a special play, or by anything big or small that you can look forward to.

Depression feeds on depression, so break the cycle. The success of everything else in this book depends on it. Depression is not permanent, but you can hasten its disappearance. Focus on your pride, your friends, your future goals, your positive surroundings. How you respond to depression is a self-fulfilling prophecy. When you believe that things will get better, they will.

COMMON PROBLEMS: PAIN, FEAR, FATIGUE, AND SEX
Pain

A survey at the Stanford Arthritis Center asked people about their concerns with arthritis. Not surprisingly, the number one concern is pain. Too often the response to this concern is "learn to live with it." This is easy to say, but hard to do. Thankfully, with a little understanding many things can be done about pain.

Pain in arthritis comes in two ways. First, the active inflammation of the disease can cause pain; most pain in rheumatoid arthritis is of this type. Second, the damaged joints can cause pain even though there is no acute inflammation; this is the kind of pain typically found in osteoarthritis. Of course you can have both kinds of pain at the same time, but usually one or the other will be the most severe.

Active pain from inflammation is best treated by reducing the inflammation, by stopping the active disease process. The anti-inflammatory drugs act on the disease process. Thus, the regular use of prescribed medication is essential to keep the pain in check. Occasionally, for very severe pain an analgesic or painkiller is needed for a short time; the painkiller might include codeine. However, while a painkiller may bring temporary relief, over a period of time it may result in addiction or may cover up the symptoms while the damage to the joint goes on.

Pain from damaged joints will usually not be helped much by medication; therefore it is important to learn nonmedical means of pain management. The following principles are important, and apply to both kinds of pain.

. We can't do two things at once. Our minds are such that we can't concentrate well on two things at the same time. Thus when you have pain it is important to keep active. Get dressed in your favorite clothes; women put on makeup, men shave. Now do something. Go to work, go out shopping, go to a movie you have wanted to see. All of these activities will make you look and feel good, and will help keep your mind off the pain. If you instead stay home in your favorite old robe and stay in bed or mope around the house you will have too much time to think about your pain and it will seem worse than it is.

. Do your exercises. Unless you are in a "flare" and have "hot" joints, your exercises will help. Some of the pain of arthritis is due to stiff, unused muscles. Therefore it is very important to keep your muscles in strong, supple condition. Muscle strength will also help keep your joints stable.

. Practice relaxation exercises. Relaxed muscles and nerve endings send out fewer pain messages and thus you have less pain.

. Don't be a martyr. Pain is individual, and it cannot be seen. Therefore, don't be afraid to tell friends and family members that you are in pain. Ask for help in carrying groceries, making beds, or mowing the lawn. Don't worry if people look at you strangely. Remember that people usually can't see your arthritis or tell that it is hurting you. A direct request for help is not being dependent, it is a direct, honest, and often necessary communication.

. Pain is closely related to stress and depression. Thus, reducing stress and depression will also reduce pain. Sometimes people are not aware of how closely attitude and pain are related. Thus, we suggest a simple exercise. For a week, keep a pain/mood diary like the one on the next page. Each day make a mark to reflect your general pain level and mood for that day. At the end of the week, connect all the pain marks and then all the mood marks. We think that you will be able to see a close connection.

Fear

People with arthritis, especially in early stages, have many fears, particularly the fear of disability or of deformity. First, you should know that most people with arthritis never have any disability or deformity. And even if you do have a mild deformity, it will very seldom be noticed by others. We see what we expect to see, and seldom notice any but the most extreme deformities. To prove this for yourself spend a day carefully observing others for deformity or disability. You will be surprised at how many you find; it is just that usually we don't notice.

PAIN/MOOD DIARY

PAIN

	SUN.	MON.	TUES.	WED.	THURS.	FRI.	SAT.
No Pain							
Terrible							

MOOD

	SUN.	MON.	TUES.	WED.	THURS.	FRI.	SAT.
Feeling Great							
Feeling Awful							

Second, don't keep your fear to yourself. Fear feeds on fear and grows into depression. Talk to someone, perhaps a friend, your doctor, or a family member. Often, talking with someone is the best thing that you can do. If you don't feel comfortable talking with any of these people, you may want to call your local health department or mental health department. Seeking help with your fears is a very healthy thing to do; the reality is never as bad as you are afraid it will be.

Fatigue

There is no question about it, arthritis can be very draining of energy. This is particularly true of rheumatoid arthritis, but it can be a problem in any type of arthritis. Thus, know that fatigue is a part of the overall problem and that you are not just imagining it. Know also that fatigue can be a sign of depression, so you should consider whether the fatigue might be lessened by treating the depression.

If the fatigue is caused by your disease then there are several things that you can do.

1. Conserve your energy (see Chapter 6 on joint protection).

2. Do the obvious—rest! Take a short nap once or twice a day. If this is impossible then just relax. Try doing a relaxation exercise.

3. Fatigue, like pain and fear, cannot be seen and is not understood by most people. Therefore tell your boss, friends, and family that fatigue is one of the problems of your arthritis and that you may have to take short rests from time to time. Gain their support in allowing you to rest. Most employers are more than willing to allow a little extra rest time for good employees. You, your family, your friends, and your employer should understand that there is a difference between fatigue and being lazy.

4. Take a good long look at yourself. Will you allow yourself to rest? Many of us build our self-images around the false ideal of being indestructible — supermom, macho man, or the perfect worker. If this is you, then reassess your position. Fatigue is one of the body's major early warning systems; it is telling you to take heed. Tune into your own body and follow its directions. The ability to rest is a strength and not a weakness.

Sex

Yes, people with arthritis, even in their seventies and eighties, actively participate in sexual activities. Somehow, when one has a disease the rest of the world thinks that they could not possibly be interested in sex, but this is not true. However, it is true that you may have to be more creative, imaginative, and flexible than most folks, and your partner may have to be more understanding. First, talk over your problems with your partner. No one wants to cause you pain, and by explaining what hurts and what doesn't you can go a long way toward more comfortable sex. Good sex includes good communication so be sure your communications are up to date. Second, try several positions until you find those most comfortable for you. Also, you may want to try other ways than intercourse of expressing sexuality. Finally, remember that there are no hard and fast rules. Beware of simplistic advice — these solutions are usually highly individual. For more information and for illustrations see some of the books listed in the Bibliography.

One final word: Sex can actually help the pain of arthritis. It seems that the excitement of sex stimulates our bodies to produce cortisone, adrenalin, and other chemicals that help to ease pain naturally; use this information as you see fit!

A note about partners of people with arthritis. Many husbands and wives have told us how hard it is to watch their spouse suffer with arthritis. They feel helpless and sometimes guilty that they can't in some way share in their partner's distress. It is hard to live with arthritis, even if you don't have it. We suggest that you talk these problems over with other partners of people with arthritis. You can find such folks through your doctor, arthritis classes, or your local Arthritis Foundation. The important thing is to know that you are not alone and that your feelings are normal.

11

What about Those Diets?

The area of foods, diet, and nutrition is one of special concern to many people with arthritis. People have many questions—"Will this food help my arthritis?" "Is there any food I should avoid?" "How can I lose weight?"—and reliable answers aren't always easy to find. In this chapter we will try to answer the basic questions and show how food and nutrition really fit into the picture.

WHAT IS "GOOD NUTRITION," ANYWAY?

To understand what is meant by good nutrition and what it has to do with good health, let us examine what is meant by the words *diet, nutrients,* and *nutrition.* Your diet is simply what you eat and drink each day. Nutrients are the many substances in your food that your body needs to work correctly. When we speak of nutrition, we mean your diet, the nutrients in it, and the whole process whereby the nutrients are used by your body. Good nutrition, then, means giving your body all the nutrients it needs, in the right amounts (not too much, not too little), when it needs them.

HOW CAN GOOD NUTRITION HELP ME?

Good nutrition helps everyone. It can help you feel fit and energetic rather than tired and weak. If you have special problems with weight or with water retention, it can help solve them. In general, good eating habits can help you feel and be as healthy and full of life as possible.

If you have arthritis, can a good diet be especially helpful? The answer is both yes and no. No special foods or diets will cure your arthritis or make it go away. However, by helping you deal with other problems (such as over-weight) and helping you feel more fit, proper nutrition can help you cope better with arthritis.

WHAT NUTRIENTS DOES MY BODY NEED?
WHY DO I NEED THEM?

Your body needs many nutrients (over 40 of them) to stay healthy. It is impractical to list all the nutrients and their uses, but the list below is a rough guide. Remember that the nutrients are spread throughout the foods we eat. No one food is "complete" or perfect, but many contain several nutrients.

BASIC NUTRIENT	PURPOSE
1. Water	Water is the "main ingredient" of your body. Water provides the proper environment for the processes that go on inside your body.
2. Carbohydrates	Carbohydrates are what we usually call sugars and starches. Carbohydrates are a main source of energy (calories). They serve as the main fuel for your body's activities.
3. Proteins	Proteins are needed for growth and for the maintenance and repair of your body's tissues (muscles, organs, bones, etc.). They also supply energy and calories.
4. Fats	Fats serve as a source of energy and as a source for certain vitamins. The fat in your body is a form of stored energy, like a reserve fuel supply.

5. Vitamins

Vitamins help control and regulate the various processes that go on in your body. Each vitamin has certain specific tasks and roles in the body, which do not change. Vitamins do *not* supply energy.

6. Minerals

Minerals help control and regulate certain body activities. They also have a role in building and repairing tissues.

7. Fiber

Fiber helps with the regulation of bowel function.

WHAT'S THE BEST WAY TO GET THE NUTRIENTS I NEED?

Just choose wisely which foods you eat. You might think that this is difficult, since there are so many nutrients. But actually, it isn't hard if you follow these guidelines.

Guideline 1. Think of calories as a "currency," like money. Depending on your size, your age, and your physical activity you have a certain number of calories you can "spend" each day on foods and still maintain a good weight. (Those of us who are fairly inactive probably have from 1500 to 2500 calories to spend each day.) With the calorie "budget" you have, you need to include all the nutrients your body needs.

If your calorie budget is small (as it is when you aren't very active, or are trying to lose weight), you need to shop around for "nutrition bargains"—foods that supply many nutrients, yet have relatively few calories. You simply can't afford to spend calories on "luxury" foods that don't provide many nutrients. If you do want an occasional luxury food, or a little more freedom from bargain hunting, you need to increase the number of calories you have to spend. The best way is to increase your physical activity.

Guideline 2. Think of the variety in your diet as your "good nutrition insurance." It is possible to eat just a few foods and have an adequate diet, but it is difficult. People whose diets are varied have a better chance of getting all the nutrients they need.

The reason variety helps is that no food gives you every nutrient, and many only give you a few. When you eat only a few foods, you may be getting a lot (even too much) of a few nutrients and very little of the rest. If you eat many different foods, you are probably getting moderate amounts of many nutrients, which is better.

Guideline 3. Think about making a few changes in your general eating habits. Most of us would be healthier if we cut down on the salt, fat, and sugar we eat and added more *complex carbohydrates*. Complex carbohydrates include fruits and vegetables, plus what we usually think of as starches (breads, cereals, grains, etc.). One benefit of these foods is that many of them (especially fruits, vegetables, and whole-grain products) provide fiber, which promotes proper bowel function. Refined sugars and sweets are not complex carbohydrates.

Many older adults cut back on fruits and vegetables because they feel that some of these cause constipation. Nothing is further from the truth. It is important to use these liberally in your diet.

Guideline 4. Keep the following Consumer's Guide to Eating in mind when you purchase, prepare, and eat your meals.

Things to Remember when Using the Consumer's Guide to Eating

1. The serving sizes and number are only a basic pattern. If you are quite active, you may need to add more food. If you are very sedentary, you may need to focus on the lower-calorie foods in each group.

2. Variety is important. Don't depend on just one or two foods in each group. Experiment a little.

3. Try not to add much fat or sugar to the foods you eat, especially if you are trying to lose weight.

4. Don't eliminate the milk products. People with arthritis still need calcium, and calcium is hard to get without dairy products.

5. Vegetables and fruits will be more nutritious if they are cooked in only a small amount of water.

6. You don't need to buy expensive foods or "health foods" to be well nourished. There are relatively inexpensive nutritious foods in every group.

7. If you are watching your food costs, it can be helpful to cut down on the number of prepared convenience foods you eat and/or eat less meat and more meat substitutes.

8. Consider using meat substitutes. Many people think that they need to eat meat every day. Actually, what they need is to get enough high-quality protein each day. Protein is composed of smaller units called *amino acids*. There are nine amino acids that your body needs but cannot make. High-quality protein is protein that contains these nine amino acids in the right proportions to meet human needs.

THE CONSUMER'S GUIDE TO EATING FOR GOOD NUTRITION

Food Group	Includes	Is a Major Source of	Approximate Serving Size	Number of Servings Needed per Day
Grains and cereals	Whole grain or enriched cereals, grains (including rice), breads, rolls, pasta, etc. (not cakes, cookies, pastries, etc.)	Carbohydrate, fiber, B vitamins	1 slice bread, or ½ cup cooked cereal or grains, or 1 oz. dry cereal (about ¾-1 cup for many cereals)	4 or more per day
Vegetables and fruits	All vegetables and fruits (pure juices may be used, but should not entirely replace whole foods) (avocados and olives are high in fat, high in calories)	Carbohydrate, fiber, iron, vitamin A, vitamin C	½ cup or 1 medium-size piece of fruit *Vitamin C* rich foods: citrus fruits, canteloupe, tomatoes, strawberries, raw cabbage, potatoes, leafy green vegetables *Vitamin A* rich foods: dark green vegetables (broccoli, kale, chard, spinach, etc.), deep yellow or orange fruits and vegetables (pumpkin, carrots, squash, apricots, sweet potatoes, etc.)	4 or more per day, including: 1 vitamin C food per day; 1 vitamin A food several times a week
Milk products	Milk (low-fat or skim preferred), cheeses (including cottage cheese), yogurt (plain has less sugar), ice cream (for occasional use) (not butter, cream, cream cheese; these are high in fat, relatively low in other nutrients)	Protein, calcium and phosphorus (minerals), riboflavin (a vitamin)	1 cup milk or yogurt, or 1-1½ oz. cheese, or 1/3 cup nonfat dry milk powder, or 1-1½ cups cottage cheese	2 or more per day
Meats and meat substitutes	Meat (preferably lean, trimmed of fat), poultry, fish, eggs, nuts (including peanut butter), legumes (dried beans and peas)	Protein, iron, B vitamins	3 oz. (excluding the bone) of cooked meat, fish, or poultry, or 2 eggs, or 4 tablespoons of peanut butter, or 1 cup dried beans or other meat substitute prepared appropriately	2 or more per day
Other foods	Fats, oils, sugar, sweets, alcohol	These foods supply few nutrients	Limit the amount eaten	You probably get more than enough without adding anything

Meat, milk, and eggs all provide high-quality protein. Most vegetables and grains don't provide high-quality protein when eaten by themselves. This is because the proportions of amino acids in plant proteins often don't match the proportions that people need. However, if several plant foods are combined properly in a meal, the body can get high-quality protein, because one food's amino acids "fill in the gaps" the other leaves.

Legumes and grains are a good example of two vegetable products that "match" or complement each other very well. Legumes (dried beans and peas) are relatively low in two amino acids that grains have plenty of, and grains are low in two amino acids that legumes can provide.

The following ten combinations of plant products will provide good, usable protein.

beans and rice	rice, soybeans, and wheat
beans and corn	peanuts, wheat, and milk
beans and wheat	peanuts, soybeans, and sesame
beans and sesame	peanuts and sunflower seeds
rice and sesame	greens and converted rice (look for the word *converted* on the package)

HOW ABOUT VITAMIN AND MINERAL SUPPLEMENTS? ARE THEY A GOOD WAY TO MAKE SURE I GET THE NUTRIENTS I NEED?

Depending on supplements is not a good idea. The five reasons for this are listed below. The same comments usually apply to cereals and other foods that are "fortified" with several vitamins and minerals.

1. Your body needs many nutrients, not just a few. When you take a supplement, you get only a few of the essential nutrients. The rest are ignored.

2. Supplements can give people a false sense of nutritional security. Some people feel that once they take their pill (or pills) they are "okay" for the day. So they don't think about the nutritive value of the foods they eat. They may end up with worse nutrition than they would have had if they hadn't taken the supplement.

3. Supplements tend to be expensive. Most people would be better off spending more on healthy foods, where money buys many nutrients, than on special supplements, where several dollars may buy only a few nutrients.

4. It is possible to get "too much of a good thing." Some vitamins and minerals build up in the body and are hard to get rid of. If people take in too much of these nutrients, health problems can result. Vitamin D is a

good example. Small amounts of the vitamin are necessary to help maintain strength in bones. But too much can cause trouble and even lead to abnormal calcium deposits in the body. Too much vitamin A can also be harmful.

5. We may not know about all the nutrients humans need yet. If you depend on supplements, you get only the nutrients that people, with current knowledge, choose to add. But if you depend on a variety of good foods, you get all the "extras" nature adds. This may be much better.

HOW CAN I USE NUTRITION AND FOODS TO HELP WITH MY ARTHRITIS?

Unless you have gout, there are no specific foods or diets that will cure or directly treat your arthritis. However, there are several things that can help you. Controlling your weight and coordinating your meals with your medications can be helpful. If so advised by your physician, restricting your salt intake may be useful. Finally, you can help yourself by learning how to critically judge "diet cures" for arthritis, so that you don't fall into any traps.

Controlling Your Weight

If you are overweight, you are putting extra loads and stress on your weight-bearing joints. This makes little sense if you have arthritis—it may make the pain or inflammation worse. Reducing your weight makes more sense—it will ease the strain, lessen the pain, improve your agility, and make you both look and feel better.

Losing weight can be a difficult task, but it is possible. If you need to reduce, perhaps this information will make the job easier.

Calories are essentially a measure of the fuel value of foods. They tell you how much work your body can do with the energy it gets when you eat a particular food. People get overweight and overfat if they eat more calories than their body needs for its activities. To lose weight and fat, they need to consume fewer calories than they use up. If, over a period of time, a person eats 3500 calories less than he or she needs, he or she will lose one pound.

There are no hard and fast rules about how to lose weight successfully, but following these steps may be helpful.

Step 1: Decide to lose weight and to change your eating habits. People are rarely successful in achieving permanent weight loss if they lack strong commitment to the idea. Check with your doctor to make sure that he or she recommends that you lose weight.

Step 2: Before you start, think about why you are overweight. Doing this may give you some clues about things you can do to help yourself. For example:

■ Some people eat too much because cooking is one of their hobbies. They enjoy eating a great deal. For them, it may help to prepare less food and to serve smaller portions.

■ Some people are overweight because they (over)eat when they get into a certain mood. They eat when they get depressed, bored, or nervous. In these cases, it may be important for people to find and plan something else to do when the mood strikes.

■ Some people eat large amounts of food almost unconsciously while they do other things. For them it is important to focus on the foods they eat, to eat slowly, and not to do anything else while they eat.

■ Some people are overweight not because they eat so much more than anyone else, but because they aren't as active. In this situation, you should try to increase your physical activity; and you also should accept the fact that you may need to regularly eat much less than others if you want to have a normal, moderate weight.

It may be easier for you to analyze your habits if you write down everything you eat for several days on a record like this:

DAY AND TIME	WHAT I ATE	HOW MUCH I ATE	WHERE I ATE	WHAT MOOD I WAS IN	WHAT I WAS DOING BESIDES EATING

Step 3: Reduce your consumption of the "luxury" foods—high-calorie foods with little nutritive value. In general, these are the foods that are not mentioned as part of the four basic groups in the Consumer's Guide to Eating.

Step 4: Use the basic foods that are lower in fat and sugar content wherever possible. Eat leaner meats, use low-fat or skim milks and cheeses. Avoid fruits canned in heavy syrup.

If necessary, eat smaller portions of the basic foods, but do not eliminate any food group. Many "low-carbohydrate" diets exclude breads and cereals as well as milk and dairy products. Do not use "crash" diets. They deprive your body of many of the nutrients it needs to be healthy, and rarely result in any long-term weight loss.

Step 5: Aim to lose weight gradually. A rate of no more than one or two pounds lost per week is best for most people. (Beware of diets that promise large, quick weight losses. With some of them, including low-carbohydrate diets, you will lose weight rapidly, but much of the loss will be water. The water will be regained quickly after you go off the diet. The aim is to lose fat, not water, so don't be deceived.)

Step 6: Don't be upset if your weight doesn't drop dramatically during the first week or if it reaches a plateau for a few weeks. When you diet, your body doesn't just burn up fat—it goes through many changes. Some of the adjustments it makes may involve changing the amount of water in your body temporarily, and this can affect your weight. But as long as you are eating less than you use up, you will be losing fat. The loss will eventually show up on the scale. If it doesn't, you are still eating too much for you. A further decrease in amount and an increase in discipline are needed.

Some additional comments on losing weight:

1. Eat slowly. When you eat slowly, you give your body time to signal you that you've eaten enough. If you eat rapidly, your body can't respond in time. By the time it tells you to stop, you've probably eaten too much.

2. Try eating small, frequent meals rather than one or two relatively large meals. This tends to help people eat less and feel more satisfied.

3. Special "dietetic" foods are not necessary. They are generally expensive and are not necessarily nutritious.

4. Try to avoid foods that contain a lot of fat or sugar and few nutrients. Sometimes you can recognize these foods because they are greasy, "rich," or very sweet. Some specific examples are:

   ■ sugar and sweets, cakes and cookies
   ■ butter, margarine, cream
   ■ gravies, sauces, dressing
   ■ fried foods
   ■ soft drinks, alcoholic beverages

5. Substitute low-calorie foods for your usual snacks and desserts. Some possibilities:

   ■ meat or vegetable broths and bouillons
   ■ vegetable soups (except cream soups)
   ■ fruits (raw or canned in their own juice)
   ■ raw vegetables, including unsweetened pickles
   ■ coffee or tea (plain)

6. Remember that no single food is necessarily "fattening" or "slimming." Since all foods have calories, eating too much of any food can make you gain weight. Moderation in your total intake is the key.

Coordinating Meals and Medications

Many of the drugs used for arthritis have some relationship to food intake and meals. Some of the drugs are best absorbed on an empty stomach. Others may cause stomach problems unless you take them with meals. When you get a new medication, check with your doctor or read Chapter 12 in this book to see whether you should take it with meals. Remember that if your physician asks you to take the drug "with every meal," he or she is probably assuming that you eat three meals a day. If you don't, be sure to tell the doctor so that any necessary adjustments can be made.

Aspirin is one example of a drug that should be taken with meals and with lots of fluids. Doing this helps prevent stomach irritation and upset.

Limiting Your Salt Intake

Salt (sodium chloride) plays many important roles in our bodies. We need sodium for our muscles and nerves to work properly. Sodium can attract and hold water, so we use it to keep the right amount of water in our bodies.

Some people, however, have too much water in their bodies. This can happen when people have high blood pressure. It can also happen when people take certain drugs, including some of those used with arthritis. In such cases, a physician may prescribe a low-sodium diet to help solve the problem.

If you have been asked to limit the amount of sodium in your diet, the following guidelines should be helpful.

1. Reduce the amount of table salt in your food.

   ■ Reduce the amount of salt used in cooking.

   ■ Don't use the salt shaker at the table.

   ■ Remember that many foods already have salt added when you buy them. Read the labels.

2. Remember that other substances besides salt contain sodium.

   ■ Become a label reader; look for the word *sodium. Sodium benzoate, sodium bicarbonate* (baking soda), and *monosodium glutamate* are examples of ingredients you may find.

3. The following foods generally contain a great deal of sodium and should be avoided.

   ■ Processed, cured, smoked, and canned meats

   ■ Salty popcorn, pretzels, crackers, nuts, potato chips, and so on

   ■ Canned soups, bouillon

   ■ Pickles, sauerkraut, and other foods treated with a brine

   ■ Some condiments, catsup, and spicy sauces (read the label)

Evaluating Diets and "Cures" for Arthritis— How to Keep from Getting Trapped

We have already mentioned that there are no known nutritional cures for arthritis. No specific foods or nutrients make arthritis better or worse, except in the case of gout. Yet, diet "cures" for arthritis appear regularly in magazines and books, and many people are interested. At the Arthritis Center we have studied the effects of diets; those who follow these fad diets do not feel any better than those who do not.

If you are interested in learning how to read articles and books on "miracle" cures so that you can judge things for yourself and not get "trapped" into unhealthy practices, this final section is for you.

Steps to Follow in Evaluating a Report of a "Cure"

Step 1: Get a copy of the book or article where the originator of the diet explains the diet and the "proof" of its effectiveness.

Step 2: Read the article, focusing on the evidence or "proof." Figure out what kind of evidence the author has. Does he or she try to persuade you with anecdotes—short stories of what happened to individual patients? Or does he or she present the results of scientific studies ("clinical trials")?

Step 3: Evaluate the evidence by asking yourself the following questions.

Questions for Anecdotes (Case Reports)

A. Get the facts.

  1. Who was involved?

  2. What was the treatment?

  3. What was the result? Were there any side effects from the treatment?

  4. What claims did the author make, based on this result?

B. Think about the facts, asking yourself:

  1. Could anything else have caused the claimed results?

   ■ Was anything besides the diet changed (medications, exercise)?

   ■ Could the change be a result of a psychological effect—"positive thinking" on the part of the patient?

   ■ Could it have been a coincidence? Arthritis pain tends to come and go.

  People often try new cures when they have the most pain, then improve and think the cure works, when it really does nothing. Usually, the improvements actually come about because the arthritis is at the "peak" of the pain cycle when he or she tries the "cure." The arthritis would improve with or without the "cure," simply because the arthritis was going into remission anyway.

  2. Were the patients different from other arthritics or from you in any important ways?

  3. If the author presents several anecdotes as evidence, are there any patterns, other than that the patient followed the diet and improved? In one currently popular book that deals with nutrition and arthritis, the author presents a number of cases in which patients followed a specific diet and improved. But if one looks closely, there is another pattern—many of the patients also lost considerable amounts of weight. This sort of thing should make you suspect that maybe it isn't the specific diet but rather the weight loss that caused the improvement.

Questions for Clinical Trials (Studies)

When you read anecdotes, you will probably find that it is difficult to answer the questions suggested above. Observations of single "cases" simply do not give enough information to tell whether treatments really work. That is the reason clinical trials are done—they help us sort out the effects of the treatment from psychological effects, coincidence, and other such things.

A clinical trial is an experiment in which one group of people gets a treatment ("Treatment X"), a similar group gets no treatment or a "traditional" treatment, and the results for the two groups are compared. If the group with the new treatment does better than the other group (the "control" group), the conclusion is that the new treatment helps. But if roughly the same proportion of people get better in both groups, the conclusion is that the new treatment has no effect or at least no more effect than the old treatment.

The following diagram may make the situation clearer. In this case, the conclusion is that Treatment X does not help, because the same number of people got better in both groups. But notice that if the researcher had only looked at the people getting Treatment X (as in case reports), he or she would probably have made the opposite (wrong) conclusion, that the treatment does help.

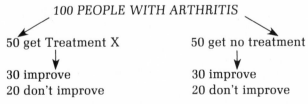

100 PEOPLE WITH ARTHRITIS

50 get Treatment X   50 get no treatment

30 improve   30 improve
20 don't improve   20 don't improve

Here are some questions to ask yourself when people present results from clinical studies.

1. Were the two groups of people really similar? If they were not, the differences between them might have confused the study, making it give deceptive results. For example, if the

group receiving no treatment has more severe arthritis, its members may not improve as much as members of the other group, whose problems are less severe. If this happens, the study may make it seem that Treatment X works better than no treatment, even though it really makes no difference. (Some things that may need to be similar in compared groups are age, sex, weight, exercise and activity patterns, and severity and type of arthritis.)

2. Were the researchers looking for a specific result? If they really wanted to prove that one group did better than the other, it may have biased them, affecting the way they saw things. ("You see what you want to see" can apply to research too, if you're not careful.)

3. Is the study published anywhere in a recent scientific journal? Editors of such magazines usually check and screen articles quite thoroughly. If a study is not published, it may mean that there are real flaws in the procedures used.

Step 4: If you are still not sure whether you should try the diet (after you evaluate the evidence), try to contact your doctor or a nutritionist to get advice.

Step 5: If you are unable to contact anyone, or if you still think that the diet may be good, ask yourself these questions:

1. Does the diet eliminate any of the basic foods or nutrients? (If so, you may well be harming your health if you follow it.)

2. Does the diet stress only a few foods, so that you will have few calories left to "spend" on the basic foods? (Again, if it does, you may be harming your health.)

3. Do the foods or supplements cost more than you can afford? (If so, following the diet may force you to cut back on other essentials, which is not good.)

4. Are you willing to put up with the trouble and expense involved, knowing that the chances are good that it won't be a cure?

If you answer no to the first three questions and yes to the last, it probably won't harm you to try the diet and see if it works for you. Remember, though, that even if it does seem to work for you, it may not work for someone else.

12
The Drug Scene
KNOW ABOUT THE MEDICATIONS THAT HELP ARTHRITIS

Knowing about your drugs is not easy. No drug is simple and a full explanation from your doctor invariably takes a lot of time. Unfortunately, that time is not always available. The interview with your doctor is an intensive experience. All too frequently discussion of the prescribed treatment serves as a quick end to the encounter. Too little time is spent on this important subject. Here, the discussions you have been having with your physician are repeated. Read the ones you need. Reread those you forget.

DRUGS TO REDUCE INFLAMMATION

The most important arthritis medicines reduce inflammation, and you have to know a little bit about this concept. Inflammation is part of the normal healing process. The body increases blood flow and sends inflammatory cells to repair wounded tissues and to kill bacterial invaders. The inflammation causes the area to be warm, red, tender, and often swollen. To understand the potential problems of drugs that reduce inflammation, it is important to recognize that inflammation is a normal process.

In rheumatoid arthritis the inflammation causes damage and thus suppression of the inflammation can be helpful in treatment. In osteoarthritis there is little inflammation or the inflammation may be necessary for the healing process. So you don't always want an anti-inflammatory drug just because you have arthritis—in rheumatoid arthritis, yes; in osteoarthritis, probably no.

Aspirin is the most important drug for arthritis. Not only is it useful itself, but it also serves as a model for understanding the benefits and problems of medical treatments for arthritis.

Aspirin is the most important drug in the world and the most misunderstood. It is among the safest drugs currently used in the United States, yet we constantly hear of its dangers. It has become downgraded by its very familiarity. Sometimes it is used as a symbol of a physician's neglect: "Take two aspirin and call me in the morning." Yet it is said to be so powerful that today the FDA would not license it if it were a new drug. The scare press reports the hazards of bleeding from the stomach or of liver damage. The same press reports the next day that aspirin may prevent heart attacks by thinning the blood. These contradictions dominate our daily encounters with aspirin.

If used properly, aspirin is a marvelous drug for many kinds of arthritis. If not used correctly, it can lead to real frustration. Read the next several paragraphs carefully; they illustrate things you need to know about aspirin specifically, but also illustrate general principles you need to know about all arthritis medications.

You must know the difference between the terms *analgesic* and *anti-inflammatory*. *Analgesic* means "pain-killing." *Anti-inflammatory* means that the redness and swelling are reduced. Aspirin provides minor pain relief and is helpful for headaches, sunburn, or other familiar problems. But it can be a major anti-inflammatory agent and can actually decrease the swelling and tissue damage in rheumatoid arthritis. Taken correctly, it is as powerful as moderate doses of cortisone.

The dosage is the difference. The pain-killing effects of aspirin are best after 2 tablets (10 grains). If you take more aspirin, you do not really get any more pain relief. You can repeat this analgesic (pain-killing) dose every 4 hours because it tends to wear off in about that time. In contrast, the anti-inflammatory activity requires high and continuous levels of aspirin in the blood. A person must take 12 to 24 tablets (5 grains each) each day and the process must be continued for 3 to 4 weeks to obtain the full effect.

This distinction is critically important. The pain-killing activity of aspirin has limited effect for major forms of arthritis. The anti-inflammatory activity is the desired effect. But this requires that the treatment be undertaken seriously, with medical supervision, and be maintained for a prolonged period. Since the effective doses are so high, most persons will encounter some side reactions and the dosage level will require adjustment. This takes us to a second consideration.

You need to know the difference between allergy and side effects. People often maintain that they cannot tolerate a drug because of problems they have had with it in the past. When the doctor asks what drugs you are allergic to, you may mention such drugs because of the problems you have had. Most of the time, you have had a side effect from the drug, not an allergy.

Allergy is relatively rare; side effects are common. Only a few people get an allergy, but everyone experiences side effects if they get enough of a drug. There are different symptoms. A skin rash, wheezing in the lungs, or a runny nose generally mean allergy. Nausea, abdominal pain, ringing in the ears, and headache usually mean side effects. If you have an allergy, that is a good reason to avoid that drug in the future. If you have side effects to a drug, usually it means that you need one or another trick to get your body to tolerate the drug better, or perhaps just a little lower dose.

These considerations are particularly important with aspirin. The treatment range is just below the level that gives side effects. So most patients receiving aspirin for anti-inflammatory purposes will have some ringing in the ears or some nausea. This is just a signal to slow down a little bit and to establish what dose is exactly the correct one for you. If you do not know this principle, you are going to give up too soon on a superb drug, and you will not get better.

You also need to know about drug absorption and drug interactions. Food delays the absorption of a medicine into your body. With some drugs the presence of food in your stomach will totally prevent the absorption of the medication. But food also protects the stomach lining and can make taking a drug more comfortable. Thus, although food may decrease the effectiveness of a medication, it also may decrease certain side effects by protecting the stomach. By and large, antacids (Maalox, Mylantin, Gelusil) act just about the same as food; they decrease absorption but protect the stomach.

Some medications are coated to protect the stomach; the coating is designed to dissolve after the tablet has passed through the stomach into the small bowel. These coatings work for some people. On occasion, the coating never dissolves and the person derives no benefit whatsoever from the drug; it passes unaltered into the toilet. On other occasions the coating doesn't last long enough and nausea is encountered anyway.

Drugs are chemicals. Interactions between two drugs (two chemicals) are extremely common. Aspirin blocks absorption from the stomach of some of the newer anti-inflammatory agents discussed in the next section. By and large, the fewer medicines you take at one time, the more predictable your response to treatment will be. Most reactions having to do with absorption or interactions with other drugs are not perfectly predictable. You may have them or you may not. The treatment for your arthritis will ultimately be unique to you. You may need to discover by trial and error some of the reactions of your own body. To figure things out, it helps if you know the final general point.

You should know about dosage equivalents, generic names, and product differences. Aspirin is huckstered more than any other drug. It is found in the drugstore in several hundred different formulations. It is "the drug doctors recommend most." Manufacturers compete to find tiny areas of difference between products that can be exploited by advertising campaigns. There are "arthritis extra-strength" aspirins, buffered aspirins, and coated aspirins. There is aspirin with extra ingredients, such as caffeine or phenacetin. There is aspirin in cold formulations with antihistamines or other compounds. There is aspirin that is advertised for its purity.

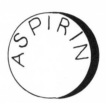

Aspirin

Color: white

A standard aspirin tablet is five grains, USP (*United States Pharmacop oeia*—the legal standard for drug strength and purity). This is 325 milligrams (mg) and the amount of drug is accurate to government standards. You always pay more for a brand-name formulation. For arthritis, do not buy aspirin that is compounded with any drugs other than possibly an antacid (Bufferin, Ascriptin). Even then, you may find it less expensive to take aspirin with an antacid such as Maalox rather than to buy buffered aspirin. You do not want the caffeine, the phenacetin, or the antihistamine ingredients. Do not use a coated aspirin (Ecotrin, Enseals) unless you have stomach problems with regular aspirin. They are more expensive and you may not get as good absorption from your stomach. All of the USP aspirins are pure enough for your use. If your body can tell a difference, stay with a product that seems to work for you. Otherwise, buy the cheapest USP aspirin that you can find. If it smells like vinegar when you open the bottle, it is too old and you should throw it out. If you have problems with the new child-proof caps, ask your pharmacist for a regular top.

The advice that follows is general advice. If your doctor's advice differs, listen to your doctor. He or she is most familiar with your specific needs. The doses and precautions listed are those known at the time of this writing and are subject to changes your doctor may know about. But if you receive advice that doesn't make sense according to the principles outlined in this section, don't hesitate to ask questions or get another opinion.

ACETYLSALICYLIC ACID (ASPIRIN)

Indications

Pain relief for osteoarthritis and local conditions such as bursitis. Anti-inflammatory agent for rheumatoid arthritis.

Dosage

For pain, two 5-grain tablets (10 grains) every four hours as needed. For anti-inflammatory action, three to four tablets, four to six times daily (with medical supervision if these doses are continued for longer than one week). The time to maximum effect is 30 minutes to one hour for pain and one to six weeks for the anti-inflammatory action.

Side Effects

Common effects include nausea, vomiting, ringing in the ears, and decreased hearing. Each of these is reversible within a few hours if the drug dosage is decreased. Allergic reactions are rare but include development of nasal polyps and wheezing. Prolonged nausea or vomiting that persists after the drug is stopped for a few days suggest the possibility of a stomach ulcer caused by the irritation of the aspirin. With an overdose of aspirin, there is very rapid and heavy breathing, and there can even be unconsciousness and coma. Be sure to keep your aspirin (and all medications) out of reach of children or visiting grandchildren.

Aspirin has some predictable effects that occur in just about everyone. Blood loss through the bowel occurs in almost all persons who take aspirin, because the blood clotting function is altered, the stomach is irritated, and aspirin acts as a minor blood-thinning agent. Up to 10 percent of those taking high doses of aspirin will have some abnormalities in the function of the liver; although these are seldom noticed by the person taking aspirin, they can be identified by blood tests. Since serious liver damage does not occur, routine blood tests to check for this complication are not required.

Special Hints

If you note ringing in the ears or a decrease in your hearing, then decrease the dose of aspirin. Your dose is just a little bit too high for the best result. If you notice nausea, an upset stomach, or vomiting, there are a variety of things you can do. First, try spreading out the dose with more frequent use of smaller numbers of pills. Perhaps instead of taking four tablets four times a day, you might take three tablets five or six times a day. Second, try taking the aspirin after meals or after an antacid, which will coat the stomach and provide some protection. Third, you can change brands and see if the nausea is related to the particular brand of aspirin you were using. Fourth, you can try coated aspirin. These are absorbed variably, but are often effective in protecting the stomach and decreasing nausea. Ecotrin is the best absorbed and Enseals is next best. Probably other brands of coated preparations should be avoided, since some of them are absorbed by very few people

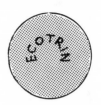

Ecotrin
5gr
Color: orange

Finally, although it is a nuisance, you can get good relief from the nausea by taking a suspension of aspirin rather than the tablet. Put the aspirin in a half glass of water and swirl it until the aspirin particles are suspended in the water. Fill another glass half full of water, drink the suspended aspirin, and wash it down with the other glass of water. This is an effective and inexpensive way to avoid nausea once you get used to the taste.

Keep track of your aspirin and always tell your doctor exactly how much you are taking. Aspirin is so familiar that sometimes we forget that we are taking a drug. Be as careful with aspirin as you would be with any drug. In particular, you may want to ask your doctor about interactions with the newer anti-inflammatory agents, with probenecid, or with blood-thinning agents, if you are taking those drugs. Pay special attention to your stomach. So many drugs cause irritation to the stomach lining that you run the risk of adding insult to injury. Two drugs that irritate the stomach lining may be more than twice as dangerous; again, the fewer medications at one time the better. Every time you talk to a doctor about drugs, be sure to describe all the drugs you are taking, not just your arthritis drugs. It is a good idea to keep a list of all the drugs you take and have it ready to show any doctor you visit, including your dentist.

TRILISATE (CHOLINE MAGNESIUM TRISALICYLATE)

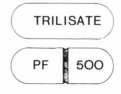

Trilisate
500mg
Color: pale orange

Purpose

To relieve pain; to reduce inflammation.

Indications

For mild pain relief of cartilage degeneration, local conditions. Also an anti-inflammatory agent for synovitis, attachment arthritis.

Dosage

For pain, one or two tablets every twelve hours. Tablets are 500 mg in size. For anti-inflammatory activity, two to three tablets each twelve hours. Each Trilisate tablet is equivalent in salicylate content to ten grains of aspirin (two usual-sized aspirin tablets). Occasionally higher doses may be needed. The maximum effect is reached in two hours for pain effects; one to six weeks are required for anti-inflammatory action to take full effect.

Side Effects

Common effects include nausea, vomiting, ringing in the ears, and decreased hearing. Each of these is reversible within a few hours if the drug dosage is decreased. Allergic reactions are rare but potentially include development of nasal polyps and wheezing. With an overdose of salicylate, there can be very rapid and heavy breathing, and even unconsciousness and coma.

Trilisate has been urged as a drug of choice in arthritis because it is much less toxic to the stomach than is aspirin. Additionally, there is less effect upon the platelets, so there is less chance of a bleeding problem. The blood salicylate level rises more slowly and lasts longer; hence, the drug does not have to be taken as often as aspirin.

But a controversy has arisen because some physicians do not believe that the anti-inflammatory activity of Trilisate is nearly as good as that of aspirin. Other physicians believe that the effects are identical. So, it seems clear that Trilisate is less toxic than ordinary aspirin, but it is not clear that it is as effective a drug. It finds particular use in patients who have had problems with stomach upset from ordinary aspirin. Trilisate does require a prescription; it is not clear why a prescription should be required for this drug any more than for regular aspirin.

Special Hints

If you note ringing in the ears or a decrease in your hearing, decrease the dose of Trilisate; it is just a little bit too high for the best results. Keep track of your Trilisate intake, and always tell the doctor exactly how much you are taking. It is possible that there may be drug interference between Trilisate and the nonsteroidal anti-inflammatory agents discussed in the following pages, so you will usually not want to take them at the same time.

Other Anti-inflammatory Agents
That Are Not Steroids

Aspirin is a *nonsteroidal anti-inflammatory agent* (NSAIA). That is, it is not a corticosteroid (like prednisone), and it is an anti-inflammatory agent because it fights inflammation. But some of the disadvantages of aspirin have been noted above. In anti-inflammatory doses, side effects such as nausea, vomiting, and ringing in the ears are common. Some persons can't tolerate these side effects. Others, either ill-advised or not persistent, don't really try. Aspirin requires many tablets and regular attention to the medication schedule. So, a class of "aspirin substitutes," given the cumbersome name of nonsteroidal anti-inflammatory agents, has been developed. In common medical usage, aspirin is not included in this group. To further simplify, we use the term *anti-inflammatory drugs* in this book. In the over-the-counter market, "aspirin substitute" usually refers to acetaminophen (Tylenol), which is discussed below as a pain reliever; acetaminophen is not an aspirin substitute for arthritis.

There is a huge market for drugs of this type. Nearly every drug company has tried to invent one and has promoted heavily whatever has been developed. Some of these drugs have been promoted in the financial pages of the newspaper or announced in press releases before the scientific evidence was complete. Clearly, you have to be careful about what you read under such circumstances. But there is some substance to the claims. Many of these drugs are good ones. They may be better for those truly unable to tolerate aspirin. Unfortunately, they are more expensive, newer, and their long-term side effects are less well known. While present evidence suggests that they are slightly safer than aspirin because of fewer stomach problems, they probably should not yet be accepted as less hazardous. Aspirin has been used for centuries and experience with these new drugs is sufficiently short that some side effects may not yet have been discovered.

In perspective, the development of these drugs represents a substantial advance. In part, this is because of the difficult problems posed by the corticosteroids (discussed in the next section). The use of the term *nonsteroidal* to distinguish these compounds underscores the importance of this feature.

In average potency, full doses of these drugs are roughly equivalent to full-dose aspirin. Gastrointestinal side effects, such as heartburn and nausea, are usually less frequent than with aspirin—hence an advantage for those with intolerant stomachs. Available evidence indicates that different drugs can be best for different individuals. These drugs come from several different chemical families and are not interchangeable. You may have to try several to find the best. The major medications in this category are discussed below in alphabetical order, according to brand name. The generic name is given in parentheses.

BUTAZOLIDINE (PHENYLBUTAZONE), TANDEARIL (OXYPHENBUTAZONE)

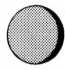

Butazolidine
100mg
Color: orange

Purpose

To reduce inflammation.

Indications

For reduction of inflammation when inflammation is causing harm, as in rheumatoid arthritis.

Dosage

Three or four 100 mg capsules spread throughout the day. Short courses of treatment given for gout or local conditions may be six capsules the first day, then five, four, three, two, and one on successive days for a six-day course.

Side Effects

Unfortunately, phenylbutazone and oxyphenbutazone can be hazardous. These were the first anti-inflammatory agents to be developed and we have had some 20 years of experience with them. We now know that on rare occasions they can cause serious problems with the blood, essentially killing all of the white cells or red cells. These conditions, termed *aplastic anemia* or *agranulocytosis*, can be fatal. They are very rare, occurring in perhaps one person in every 10,000. When encountered, the conditions are sometimes reversible after the drug is stopped, and they don't seem to occur if the drug is used only for a short period. Because of this toxicity, most doctors use the other drugs described below in preference to Butazolidine. This may be unfortunate, since Butazolidine is a very effective medication in many instances.

Irritation of the stomach lining may also occur, with nausea, heartburn, indigestion, and occasionally vomiting. Some persons retain fluid with Butazolidine and a low-salt diet is recommended. Allergic reactions, including rash, are rare.

Special Hints

For nausea, spread the dose out a little through the day and take the capsules on a full stomach, perhaps one-half hour after meals. If you don't have a meal at that time, take an antacid half an hour before the medication. Occasionally, some people will have better luck with Tandearil if stomach upset with Butazolidine is a major problem. Watch your weight; if it goes up you are probably retaining fluid. If so, reduce the salt in your diet (see Chapter 11), and be alert for any signs of shortness of breath. If shortness of breath occurs, call the doctor without delay.

While you are taking this drug, blood counts are recommended by most doctors, even though these tests do not protect you against the bad reaction. Possibly, however, they may enable an adverse reaction to be discovered more quickly. Blood counts every two weeks for the first three months and once a month thereafter are recommended by many doctors. For a short six-day course, no blood tests are required by most doctors. You should be able to tell if this is going to be a good drug for you within one week. If you haven't noticed major benefit, you may want to discuss a change in medication with your doctor.

CLINORIL (SULINDAC)

Clinoril (Sulindac)
150mg and 200mg

Color: bright yellow

Purpose

To reduce inflammation, to reduce pain slightly.

Indications

For anti-inflammatory action and mild pain relief.

Dosage

One 150 mg tablet twice a day. This drug also comes in a 200 mg tablet and dosage may be increased to 200 mg twice a day if needed. Maximum recommended dose is 400 mg a day.

Side Effects

Gastrointestinal side effects, with irritation of the stomach lining, are the most common, and include nausea, indigestion, and heartburn. Stomach pain has been reported in ten percent of subjects, and nausea, diarrhea, constipation, headache, and rash in from three to nine percent. Ringing in the ears, fluid retention, itching, and nervousness have been reported. A few persons have had bleeding from the stomach. Allergic reactions are rare. The use of aspirin in combination with this drug is not recommended by the manufacturer, since aspirin apparently decreases absorption from the intestine.

Special Hints

Sulindac has no particular advantages or disadvantages compared with the other anti-inflammatory agents described in this section. At this writing, Clinoril is the most expensive of these agents. It has been promoted beyond its worth as a "miracle" agent; new drugs are not necessarily improvements.

For stomach upset, take the pills after meals; skip a dose or two if necessary. Antacids may be used for gastrointestinal problems and may sometimes help. Check with your doctor if the distress continues. Maximum therapeutic effect is achieved after about six weeks of treatment, but you should be able to see a major effect in the first week if Clinoril is going to be a really good drug for you.

FELDENE (PIROXICAM)

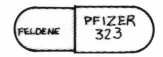

Feldene
20mg

Color: dark red

Purpose

To reduce inflammation; to reduce pain slightly.

Indications

For anti-inflammatory activity and mild pain in rheumatoid arthritis, local conditions, and sometimes cartilage degeneration (osteoarthritis).

Dosage

One 20 mg tablet once daily. Do not exceed this dosage. This is a long-acting drug, and it need be taken only once daily.

Side Effects

The drug has been generally well tolerated, although gastrointestinal symptoms including irritation of the stomach lining do still occur, as well as nausea, indigestion, and heartburn. Allergic reactions, including skin rashes or asthma, are very rare. Peptic ulceration can occur, particularly if the recommended dosage is exceeded. Fluid retention is only very occasionally a problem.

Special Hints

Since this is a long-acting drug, some seven to twelve days are required before the benefits are apparent, and full benefits may not be clear until six weeks or more. Aspirin should be avoided in general. Dosage recommendations and indications for use in children have not been established. Some patients with rheumatoid arthritis or osteoarthritis prefer Feldene, particularly because of its relatively mild gastrointestinal toxicity and because of the convenience of once-a-day dosage. On the other hand, there has been no long-term experience with the drug, and it is felt to be a symptomatic medication rather than one that might alter the underlying disease.

INDOCIN (INDOMETHACIN)

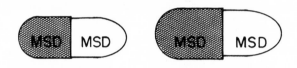

Indocin
25mg and 50mg
Color: blue/white

Purpose

To reduce inflammation, to slightly reduce pain.

Indications

For reduction of inflammation and for mild pain relief.

Dosage

One 25 mg capsule three to four times daily. For men or large women, doses totaling as high as 150 to 200 mg (six to eight capsules) may be required and tolerated each day. It is also available in 50 mg capsules.

Side Effects

Irritation of the stomach lining, including nausea, indigestion, and heartburn, occurs with a number of people. Allergic reactions (including skin rash or asthma) are very rare. The biggest problem is headache and a bit of a goofy feeling reported by some patients. This problem often goes away after two or three weeks but can be a good reason to switch to another nonsteroidal drug if it is troublesome.

Special Hints

Many doctors find Indocin to be rather weak for treatment of rheumatoid arthritis in early stages, although it is sometimes effective in later stages. In a long-term illness, maximum effect may take six weeks or so, but you should be able to tell within one week if it is going to be a major help. This is the cheapest of the new nonsteroidal drugs, so if it works you may save money.

There are some problems with absorption of Indocin from the intestine. If you take it after meals, you have less stomach irritation, but some people do not absorb the drug very well. So for maximum effect you need to take it on an empty stomach and for maximum comfort to take it on a full stomach. Trial and error may be necessary to establish the best regimen for you. Aspirin poses another problem. When some individuals take aspirin with Indocin, the Indocin is not absorbed from the intestine. Usually you will not want to take these two drugs together, since you will get more irritation of the stomach lining but no more therapeutic effect than if you just took the aspirin. If this drug makes you feel mentally or emotionally fuzzy for more than the first few weeks, we think that is a good reason to discuss a change in medication with your doctor.

MECLOMEN (MECLOFENAMATE)

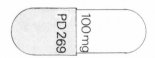

Meclomen (Meclofenamate sodium)
100mg

Color: orange/off white

Purpose

To reduce inflammation; to reduce pain slightly.

Indications

For anti-inflammatory action in attachment arthritis, synovitis, local conditions, and occasionally with degenerative cartilage changes.

Dosage

The total daily dosage is 200 to 400 mg, usually administered in three or four equal doses. The drug is supplied in 50 mg and 100 mg capsules.

Side Effects

Gastrointestinal side effects are most commonly reported and include diarrhea in approximately one-quarter of patients, nausea in 11 percent, and other gastrointestinal problems in 10 percent. Over the long term, at least one-third of patients will have at least one episode of diarrhea. The diarrhea is sufficiently severe to require discontinuation of treatment in approximately 4 percent of patients. A variety of other generally minor side effects have been reported but do not appear to be at all common.

Special Hints

This drug was introduced only in 1980, and there is relatively little experienc with it. It is probably comparable in effectiveness to the other nonsteroida agents. It is not yet recommended for children, and its effects have not bee studied in patients with very severe rheumatoid arthritis. It may be take with meals or milk to control gastrointestinal complaints. Maximum effect i achieved after about six weeks of treatment, but you should be able to see major effect in the first week if it is going to be a really good drug for you Avoidance of aspirin and other medications while taking this drug is advisabl but not essential.

MOTRIN AND RUFEN (IBUPROFEN)

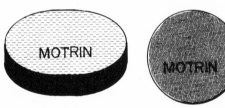

Motrin

Color: 600mg — yellow
        400mg — red-orang

Motrin and Rufen are the same drug, ibuprofen, produced by two differer companies.

Purpose

To reduce inflammation, to slightly reduce pain.

Indications

For anti-inflammatory action and mild pain relief.

Dosage

One or two 400 mg tablets three times daily. Maximum daily recommende dosage is 2400 mg, or six tablets.

Side Effects

Gastrointestinal side effects, with irritation of the stomach lining, are th most common, and include nausea, indigestion, and heartburn. Allergi reactions are rare and the drug is generally well tolerated. A very fe individuals have been observed who have had *aseptic meningitis* apparentl related to this drug. Here, the person experiences headache, fever, and sti neck, and examination of the spinal fluid shows an increase in the protei and cells. The syndrome resolves when the drug is stopped, but can come back again if the drug is given again. Occasionally, individuals may retain fluid with this medication.

Special Hints

Motrin is not consistently useful for the treatment of rheumatoid arthritis. Overall, many doctors are beginning to feel that it is one of the weaker therapeutic agents in this group. If you are not getting enough relief from it, you may wish to discuss a change in medication with your doctor. Avoidance of aspirin and other medications while taking Motrin is advisable but not essential. It is absorbed reasonably well even on a full stomach, so if you have problems with irritation of the stomach take the drug after an antacid or after a meal. Maximum effect is achieved after about six weeks of treatment, but you should be able to see a major effect in the first week if it is going to be a really good drug for you.

NALFON (FENOPROFEN)

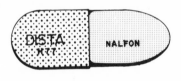

Nalfon

Color: 300mg — dark yellow/yellow
        600mg — orange-yellow

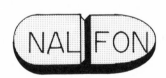

Purpose

To reduce inflammation, to slightly reduce pain.

Indications

For anti-inflammatory activity and mild pain relief in rheumatoid arthritis, local conditions, and sometimes cartilage degeneration (osteoarthritis).

Dosage

One or two 300 mg capsules three or four times a day. Maximum recommended dosage is ten tablets daily. It is now available in 600 mg capsules, with a maximum dosage of five tablets daily.

Side Effects

Irritation of the stomach lining is the most frequent side effect and includes nausea, indigestion, and heartburn. Allergic reactions including skin rash or asthma are very rare. Fluid retention is only very occasionally a problem.

Special Hints

For stomach irritation, reduce the dose, spread it out more throughout the day, or take the drug after meals or after antacid. Maximum effect may take six weeks or more, but you should see major benefit in the first week if the drug is going to be a great help to you. Aspirin should be avoided in general although the evidence for its effect on the absorption of Nalfon is controversial. Nalfon is quite useful in rheumatoid arthritis and is preferred by many individuals to aspirin on the basis of better effect on the disease as well as less bothersome side effects. It has found uses in osteoarthritis, particularly of the hip.

NAPROSYN (NAPROXEN)

Naprosyn
250mg

Color: light yellow

Purpose

To reduce inflammation, to slightly reduce pain.

Indications

For anti-inflammatory action and mild pain relief.

Dosage

One 250 mg tablet two or three times a day. Maximum recommended dosage is 750 mg (three tablets) a day.

Side Effects

Gastrointestinal side effects, with irritation of the stomach lining, are the most common, and include nausea, indigestion, and heartburn. Skin rash and other allergic problems are very rare. Fluid retention has been reported in a few individuals.

Special Hints

Naprosyn has an advantage over other drugs of this class in having a longer "half-life." Thus, you do not have to take as many tablets as with the other medicines in this group. Each tablet lasts from 8 to 12 hours. In general, aspirin should be avoided, since it interferes with Naprosyn in some individuals. If you notice fluid retention, reduce your salt intake (see Chapter 11), and discuss a change in medication with your doctor. Naprosyn is liked by many people because of the small number of tablets required. It is quite effective in rheumatoid arthritis and is preferred by some people over aspirin and other drugs of this group. Degenerative arthritis of the hip also responds. If you have stomach irritation, try taking the tablets on a full stomach or after antacids. Although absorption may be slightly decreased, you may be more comfortable overall.

RUFEN (IBUPROFEN)

See Motrin.

Rufen
400mg

Color: bright pink

TOLECTIN (TOLMETIN SODIUM)

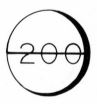

Tolectin
200mg

Color: white

Purpose

To reduce inflammation, to reduce pain slightly.

Indications

For anti-inflammatory action and mild pain relief.

Dosage

Two 200 mg tablets three or four times daily. Maximum recommended dosage is 2000 mg, or ten tablets daily. Larger tablet sizes may soon be available.

Side Effects

The most frequent side effects are gastrointestinal, as with other drugs (this group. Irritation of the stomach lining can cause nausea, heartburn, and indigestion. Occasionally, individuals note fluid retention. Allergic reaction such as rash or asthma are very rare.

Special Hints

For irritation of the stomach, decrease the dose or spread the tablets ov throughout the day. Absorption will be slightly decreased if you take the dru after meals or after antacids, but greater comfort may result. Aspirin an other drugs of this class may potentially interfere with absorption and th best rule is to take just one drug at a time. Tolectin is useful in rheumatoi arthritis. It has found use in degenerative arthritis of the hip and for trea ment of local conditions. As with other drugs of this group, certain individua will prefer Tolectin to all other drugs of the group.

Corticosteroids (Prednisone)

In about 1950, a widely heralded miracle occurred—the introduction of cort sone for the treatment of arthritis. The Nobel prize was awarded to th doctors who developed this drug. Persons with rheumatoid arthritis an other forms of synovitis suddenly noted that the swelling and pain in thei joints decreased and that the overall toxicity of the disease disappeare They felt fine.

The initial enthusiasm for cortisone in arthritis was tremendous. Bu over the following years, a number of major cautions began to be voice Slowly, the cumulative side effects of the cortisonelike drugs began to b recognized. For many individuals, the side effects were clearly greater tha any benefits obtained. Cortisone became the model of a drug that provide early benefits but late penalties. Now, with a quarter of a century experience with these drugs, our perspective is more complete. They repr sent a major treatment for arthritis, but their use is appropriate in only relatively small number of cases and then only with full attention to potenti complications.

Steroids are natural hormones manufactured by the adrenal gland When used medically, they are given in doses somewhat higher than th amounts the body generally makes. In these doses they suppress the functic of your own adrenal glands and lead to a kind of drug dependency as th gland slowly shrinks. After many months of steroid use, the drug must b withdrawn slowly to allow your own adrenal gland to return to full functio otherwise an "adrenal crisis" can occur in which you just don't have enoug hormone. Steroids must be taken exactly as directed and a physician's clos advice is always required.

Let's discuss the side effects. They can be divided into categories depending upon the length of time you have been taking the steroid and the dose prescribed. Side effects result from a combination of how high the dose and how long you have been taking it. If you have been taking steroids for less than one week, side effects are quite rare even if the dose has been high.

If you have been taking high doses for one week to one month, you are at risk for development of ulcers, mental changes including psychosis or depression, infection with bacterial germs, or acne over the skin. The side effects of steroid treatment become most apparent after one month to one year of medium to high dosage. The individual becomes fat in the central parts of the body, with a buffalo hump on the lower neck and wasting of the muscles in the arms and legs. Hair growth increases over the face, skin bruises appear, and stretch marks develop over the abdomen. After years of steroid treatment (even with low doses) there is loss of calcium, resulting in fragile bones. Fractures can occur with only slight injury, particularly in the spine. Cataracts slowly develop and the skin becomes thin and translucent. Some physicians believe that hardening of the arteries occurs more rapidly and that there may be complications of inflammation of the arteries.

Many of these side effects will occur in everyone who takes sufficient doses of cortisone or its relatives for a sufficient period of time. The art of managing arthritis with corticosteroids involves knowing how to minimize these side effects. The physician will work with you to keep the dose as low as possible at all times. If possible, you may be instructed to take the drug only once daily rather than several times daily, since there are fewer side effects when it is taken this way. If you are able to tolerate the drug only every other day, this is even better, for the side effects are then quite minimal. Unfortunately, many people find that the dosage schedules that cause the fewest side effects also give them the least relief.

Steroids are always to be used with great respect and caution. Some experienced doctors still use low-dose corticosteroid treatment in rheumatoid arthritis, demonstrating that the proper indications for use of these drugs is somewhat controversial. High-dose cortisone treatment for uncomplicated rheumatoid arthritis has long been considered bad practice in the United States; it remains the essence of some quack treatments of arthritis, such as those available in Mexican border towns. Corticosteroids are harmful in infectious arthritis and should not be given by mouth in local conditions or in osteoarthritis.

There are three ways to give corticosteroids. They can be taken by mouth, they can be given by injection into the painful area, or an injection of adrenal cortical stimulating hormone (ACTH) can be given to cause an individual's own adrenal gland to increase production of hormones. Prednisone (or prednisolone) is the steroid usually given by mouth and is the reference steroid discussed here. There are perhaps 20 different steroid drugs now available. Cortisone itself retains too much fluid and the second

drug developed, hydrocortisone, has the same deficit. The fluorinated ste
oids, such as triamcinolone, cause greater problems with muscle wastir
than does prednisone. The steroids sold by brand name are about 20 times $\;$
expensive as prednisone and do not have any major advantages. Hence, the
is little reason to use any of these other compounds for administration $\;$
steroids by mouth. Use prednisone.

PREDNISONE

Prednisone
5mg

Color: white

Purpose

To reduce inflammation, to suppress immunological responses.

Indications

For suppression of serious systemic manifestations of connective tissu
disease, such as kidney involvement. Occasionally, for use in suppressing th
inflammation of rheumatoid arthritis.

Dosage

The normal body makes the equivalent of about 5 to 7.5 mg of prednisor
each day. "Low-dose" prednisone treatment is from 5 to 10 mg. A "modera
dose" ranges from 15 to 30 mg per day and a "high dose" from 40 to 60 mg p
day, or even higher. The drug is often most effective when given in sever
doses throughout the day, but side effects are least when the same total dai
dose is given as infrequently as possible.

Side Effects

Prednisone causes all of the side effects of the corticosteroids listed abov
Allergy is extremely rare. Side effects are related to dose and to duration $\;$
treatment. The side effects are major and include fatal complication
Psychological dependency often occurs and complicates efforts to get off th
drug once you have begun.

Special Hints

Discuss the need for prednisone very carefully with your doctor befo
beginning. The decision to start steroid treatment for a chronic disease is

major one and you want to be sure that the drug is essential. You may want a second opinion if the explanation does not completely satisfy you. When you take prednisone, follow your doctor's instructions very closely. With some drugs it does not make much difference if you start and stop them on your own, but prednisone must be taken extremely regularly and exactly as prescribed. You will want to help your doctor decrease your dose of prednisone whenever possible, even if this does cause some increase in your symptoms.

A funny thing happens when you reduce the dose of prednisone; a syndrome called *steroid fibrositis* can cause increased stiffness and pain for a week or ten days after each dose reduction. Sometimes this is interpreted as return of the arthritis and the opportunity to reduce the dose of prednisone is lost. If you are going to take prednisone for a long time, ask your doctor about taking some vitamin D along with it. There is some evidence, still controversial, that the loss of bone, the most critical long-term side effect, can be reduced if you take vitamin D.

If you are having some side effects, ask your doctor about once-a-day or every-other-day use of the prednisone. Watch your salt intake and keep it low, since there is a tendency to retain fluid with prednisone. Watch your diet as well, since you will be fighting an increase in appetite and a tendency to put on unseemly fat. If you stay active and limit the calories you take in, you can minimize many of the ugly side effects of the steroid medication and can improve the strength of the bones and the muscles. If you are taking a corticosteroid other than prednisone by mouth, ask your physician if it is all right to switch to the equivalent dose of prednisone. (See Chapter 11 for further hints on nutrition.)

STEROID INJECTIONS (DEPO-MEDROL, MANY OTHERS)

Purpose

To reduce inflammation in a local area.

Indications

Noninfectious inflammation and pain in a particular region of the body. Or a widespread arthritis with one or two areas causing most of the problem.

Dosage

Dosage varies depending upon the preparation and purpose desired. The frequency of injection is more important. Usually injections should not be repeated more frequently than every six weeks and a limit of three injections in a single area is observed by many physicians.

Side Effects

Steroid injections resemble a very short course of prednisone by mouth and therefore have few side effects. They result in a high concentration of the steroid in the area that is inflamed and can have quite a pronounced effect in reducing this inflammation. If a single area is injected many times, the injection appears to cause damage in that area. This has resulted in serious problems in frequently injected areas, such as the elbows of baseball pitchers. Some studies suggest that as few as ten injections can cause increased bone destruction; hence most doctors stop injecting well before this time.

Special Hints

If one area of your body is giving you a lot of trouble, an injection frequently makes sense. The response to the first injection will tell you quite accurately how much sense it makes. If you get excellent relief that lasts for many months, reinjection is indicated if the problem returns. The steroid injections contain a "long-acting" steroid, but it is in the body for only a few days. The effects may last much longer than this, however, since a cycle of inflammation and injury may be broken by the injection. If you get relief for only a few days, then injection is not going to be a very useful treatment for you. If you get no relief at all or an increase in pain, this is an obvious sign that other kinds of treatment should be sought. If you can find a "trigger point" on your body where pressure reproduces your major pain, then injection of this trigger point is frequently beneficial. Occasionally, persons with osteoarthritis get benefit from injections, but injections are usually not helpful unless there is inflammation in the area.

Gold Salts and Penicillamine

These are major-league drugs, although no one knows exactly why they are so effective in so many individuals. They provide dramatic benefits to over two-thirds of persons with severe rheumatoid arthritis. Each has major side effects that require stopping treatment for at least one-quarter of the users and that may in rare cases be fatal. Gold salts and penicillamine are two very different kinds of drugs, but there are striking similarities in the type and magnitude of good effects and in the type of side effects. Neither appears to be of use in any category other than rheumatoid arthritis, but the scientific proof of their effectiveness in RA is impressive.

These agents can result in remission of the arthritis. In perhaps one quarter of users the disease will actually be so well controlled that neither doctor nor patient can find any evidence of it. Usually these drugs have to be continued in order to maintain the remission, but the effects can be more dramatic than with any other agent to reduce inflammation, except possibly

ome of the more dangerous immunosuppressant drugs. Individuals who use
ıese drugs must accept certain significant hazards, but there is a good
hance of very major benefit. In rheumatoid arthritis, these drugs have been
roven to retard the process of joint destruction.

If you are not able to tolerate one of these drugs, you may be able to
ılerate the other. If you don't get a good response from one, you may from
ıe other. After failure with one drug, the chances decrease a little, but
uccess with the second drug is still common.

Which should be used first? No one knows. In England, penicillamine is
sually used first. In the United States, it is gold. Gold must be given by
ıjection and requires a visit to the doctor every week for a while. With costs
f blood tests, the total dollar cost of the initial course may be $800 or more.

Penicillamine can be taken by mouth, and while the drug itself is
xpensive, the total cost may be less. In terms of effectiveness and in risk,
ou can consider these two drugs about the same.

ÍOLD SALTS (MYOCHRISINE, SOLGANOL)

³urpose

'o reduce inflammation.

ndications

ₕeumatoid arthritis that is not responsive to less hazardous medications or
s severe and rapidly progressive.

³osage

i0 mg per week by intramuscular injection for 20 weeks, then one to two
ınjections per month thereafter. Many doctors use smaller doses for the first
wo injections to test for allergic reactions to the injections. Sometimes
loctors will give more or less than this standard dosage depending upon your
ıody size and response to treatment. "Maintenance" gold treatment refers to
ınjections after the first 20 weeks (which result in about 100 mg of total gold).
¯he dosage and duration of maintenance therapy varies quite a bit; with good
ᵉsponses, the gold maintenance may be continued for many years, with
ınjections given every two to six weeks. Maintenance dosage may be much
ower—from 10 to 25 mg. The duration is more important than the dosage.

Side Effects

Τhe gold salts accumulate very slowly in the tissues of the joints and in other
ɔarts of the body. Hence, side effects usually occur only after a considerable

amount of gold has been received, although allergic reactions can occur even with the initial injection. The major side effects have to do with the skin, the kidneys, and the blood cells. The skin may develop a rash, usually occurring after ten or more injections, with big red spots or blotches, often itchy. If the rash remains a minor problem, the drug may be cautiously continued, but occasionally a very serious rash occurs following gold injections.

The kidney can be damaged so that protein leaks out of the body through the urine. This is called *nephrosis* or the *nephrotic syndrome* if it is severe. When it is recognized and the drug is stopped, the nephrosis usually goes away, but cases have been reported in which it did not reverse. The blood cell problems are the most dangerous. They can affect either the white blood cells or the platelets, those blood cells that control the clotting of the blood. In each case, the gold causes the bone marrow to stop making the particular blood cell. If the white cells are not made, the body becomes susceptible to serious infections that can be fatal. If the platelets are not made, the body is subject to serious bleeding episodes that can be fatal. These problems almost always reverse when the drug is stopped, but reversal may take a number of weeks, during which time the person is at risk for a major medical problem.

There are other side effects, such as ulcers in the mouth, a mild toxic effect on the liver, or nausea, but they usually are not as troublesome. Overall, about one-quarter of users have to stop their course of treatment because of the side effects. One or two percent of users experience significant side effect; the other users don't really notice very much of a problem, even though a serious side effect may be about to occur. Less than one in a thousand times there may be a fatal side effect. With careful monitoring, the drug is reasonably safe and its benefits justify its use, since over 70 percent of those treated with gold show moderate or marked improvement. However, you must maintain your respect for this treatment and keep up regular blood tests to detect early side effects. One final note: Most side effects occur during the first initial period of 20 injections. Serious side effects during the maintenance period are unusual.

Special Hints

You must learn to be patient with gold treatment. The gold accumulates slowly in the body and responses are almost never seen in the first 10 weeks of treatment. Improvement begins slowly after that and major improvement usually evident by the end of 1000 mg, or 20 weeks. Similarly, if the drug stopped, it requires many months before the effect is totally lost. In one famous study, the gold group was still doing better than the control group two years after the drug had been stopped, although most of the effect of the drug had been lost by that time. After a side effect, many doctors will suggest that the drug be tried again. Often, this can be worthwhile if the approach very cautious, since the drug is frequently tolerated the second time around. At the Arthritis Center we do not try gold salts again if there has been a problem with the blood, but we will use it again cautiously after mild skin reactions or mild amounts of protein loss through the urine.

To minimize the chance of serious side effects, most doctors recommend that a check be made of the urine for protein leakage, of the white cells and the platelets, and that the patient is questioned about skin rash before every injection. This is good practice. Unfortunately, the combination of 20 doctor visits, 20 injections, 20 urinalyses, 20 blood counts, and so forth, makes the cost of initiating gold treatment approximately $800 when pursued in this manner. There are some ways to decrease this cost while preserving the safety. You can ask your doctor to prescribe some test kits so that you can test your urine for protein at home. This is a very easy technique. You can ask if it is possible to have just a platelet smear and a white count rather than a complete blood count each time. You can inquire whether it is possible to have the nurse give an injection after checking the blood count without actually having a doctor visit every week. And, some people have successfully been given their own shots at home with the help of their family, although this is not acceptable to many. By using such techniques, you can save half to three-quarters of the cost of a course of gold treatment.

RIDAURA (AURANOFIN)

Purpose

To reduce inflammation in rheumatoid arthritis.

Indications

For anti-inflammatory activity in rheumatoid arthritis.

Dosage

Average dosage is 6 mg daily. The drug is slowly absorbed and distributed through the body, and weeks to months may be required before full therapeutic effect is achieved. This drug appears closely similar to intramuscular gold injections in effectiveness, and the mechanism of action is probably the same. Side effects are much reduced compared to those of intramuscular gold injections.

Side Effects

The most common side effect is dose-related diarrhea, which occurs at some time in approximately one-third of treated patients but requires discontinuation in only about 2 percent of patients. Skin rash has occurred in 4 percent, mild kidney problems in 1 percent, and problems with the platelets in half of 1 percent of patients.

Special Hints

This drug is useful in rheumatoid arthritis, for which it may be a very important drug. It is not believed to be effective in osteoarthritis, gout, or minor rheumatic conditions. It may or may not have an eventual role in psoriatic arthritis, ankylosing spondylitis, and the arthritis of children. If diarrhea is encountered, the dose should be reduced. As with intramuscular gold injections, patients should be monitored periodically for blood complications, skin rash, and protein loss in the urine. Follow your doctor's advice for the particular tests required and the frequencies with which they are needed. This is a powerful drug and needs to be used with respect.

PENICILLAMINE (CUPRIMINE)

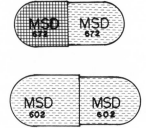

Penicillamine (Cuprimine)

Color: 125mg—gray/yellow
        250mg—yellow

Purpose

To reduce inflammation.

Indications

Rheumatoid arthritis that is not responsive to less hazardous medications or is severe and rapidly progressive.

Dosage

Usually 250 mg (one tablet or two 125 mg tablets) per day for one month, then two tablets (500 mg) a day for one month, then three tablets (750 mg) per day for one month, and finally four tablets (1000 mg) per day. Dosage is usually not increased rapidly, and may be increased even more slowly than this. After remission, the drug can be continued indefinitely, usually at a reduced dosage. And if a good result is obtained earlier, you can stop with the lower dose.

Side Effects

These closely parallel those noted above for gold injections. The major side effects are skin rash, protein leakage through the urine, or a decrease in production of the blood cells. Additionally, individuals may have nausea, and some notice a metallic taste in their mouth or a decreased sense of taste. Penicillamine weakens the connective tissue so that the healing of a cut is delayed, and a scar may not have the same strength it would have without the penicillamine. So, stitches following a cut should be left in for a longer period of time, and wound healing should be expected to be delayed. Surgery under these circumstances may be more difficult.

Special Hints

Penicillamine takes a number of months to reach its full therapeutic effect and the effect persists for a long time after you stop taking the drug. Responses usually take from three to six months but can be as late as nine months after the drug is begun. Because of the risk of side effects, doctors have now adopted the "go low, go slow" approach given in the dosage schedule above. When full doses were begun earlier, the frequency of side effects was higher. Even now, only about three-quarters of individuals will complete the treatment and the remainder will have some side effects, approximately the same as those listed for gold salts. The drug may be tried again after a side effect if the side effect has been mild. We do not try the drug again if there has been a problem with the blood counts, but may cautiously try it if there has been a minor problem with protein in the urine, a minor skin rash, or minor nausea.

Monitoring for side effects has to be carefully performed. Usually a blood count or smear, a urinalysis for protein leakage, and questioning of the person about side effects are required every two weeks or even more frequently. It should be noted that with both penicillamine and gold, careful monitoring improves your chances of not having a serious side effect, but does not eliminate them. These drugs contain an intrinsic hazard that no physician can eliminate. Again, you can negotiate to have some of the drug monitoring done by a local laboratory and review the results yourself, check your own urine for protein, and so forth, if you desire. Most doctors who use these drugs a good deal have evolved some method of minimizing the cost of the monitoring. Again, after the first six months, side effects are relatively rare but still do occur. Some individuals will have an excellent response to the penicillamine, even though they never get up to the full dosage of 1000 mg per day.

DRUGS TO REDUCE PAIN

This section is included mainly to emphasize that pain-reducing drugs have little place in the treatment of arthritis. Consider their four major disadvantages. First, they don't do anything for the arthritis, they just cover it up. Second, they help defeat the pain mechanism that tells you when you are doing something that is injuring your body. If you suppress it, you may injure your body without being aware of it. Third, the body adjusts to pain medicines, so that they aren't very effective over the long term. This phenomenon is called *tolerance* and develops to some extent with all of the drugs we commonly use. Fourth, pain medicines can have major side effects. The side effects range from stomach distress to constipation to mental changes. Most of these drugs are "downers," which you don't need if you have arthritis. You need to be able to cope with a somewhat more difficult living situation than the average person. These drugs decrease your ability to solve problems.

Many individuals develop a tragic dependence on these agents. In arthritis, the addiction is somewhat different from what we usually imagine. Most persons with arthritis are not truly addicted to codeine or Percodan or Demerol. They are psychologically dependent on these drugs as a crutch and become inordinately concerned with an attempt to eliminate every last symptom. These agents conflict with the attempt to achieve independent living.

By and large, use these drugs only for the short term and only when resting the sore part, so that you don't reinjure it while the pain is suppressed. Drugs mentioned first in this list are less harmful than those listed later. Drugs to reduce inflammation, discussed above, may reduce pain through direct pain action as well as through reduction of inflammation. This is preferable.

These same principles hold for a number of less common pain relievers not described in the following section.

ACETAMINOPHEN (TYLENOL, OTHER BRANDS)

Tylenol
325mg

Color: white

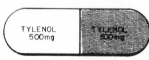
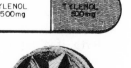

Extra-Strength Tylenol
500mg

Color: tablet—white
      capsule—white/red

Purpose

For temporary relief of minor pain.

Indications

Mild temporary pain, particularly with cartilage degeneration (osteoarthritis).

Dosage

Two tablets (ten grains) every four hours as needed.

Side Effects

Minimal. Unlike aspirin, acetaminophen usually does not upset the stomach, does not cause ringing in the ears, does not affect the clotting of the blood, does not interact with other medications, and is about as safe as can be. Of course, as with any drug, there are occasional problems, but this drug is frequently recommended in place of aspirin for children because of its greater safety. And acetaminophen is the only drug in this category that is not addictive.

Special Hints

Acetaminophen is not anti-inflammatory; thus it is not an aspirin substitute in the treatment of arthritis. If the condition is not an inflammatory one, then it may be approximately as useful as aspirin with fewer side effects. It is only a mild pain reliever and therefore has fewer disadvantages than the following agents. It is relatively inexpensive. Advertised names, such as Tylenol, may be more expensive than other acetaminophens.

DARVON (DARVON COMPOUND, DARVO-TRAN, DARVOCET, DARVOCET-N, PROPOXYPHENE)

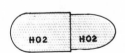 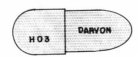

Darvon

32mg and 65mg

Color: pink

Purpose

Mild pain relief.

Indications

For short-term use in decreasing mild pain.

Dosage

One-half grain (32 mg) or one grain (65 mg) every four hours as needed for pain.

Side Effects

These drugs are widely promoted and widely used with a reasonably good safety record. In some cases, side effects may be due to the aspirin or other medication in combination with the Darvon. Most worrisome to us has been the mentally dull feeling that many individuals report, often described as a gray semiunhappy fog. Others do not seem to notice this effect. Side reactions include dizziness, headache, sedation, somnolence, paradoxical excitement, skin rash, and gastrointestinal disturbances.

Special Hints

Darvon is not anti-inflammatory and is thus not an aspirin substitute. The pain relief given is approximately equal to aspirin in most cases. The drug is more expensive than aspirin or acetaminophen. It can induce dependence, particularly after long-term use.

CODEINE (EMPIRIN #1, 2, 3, 4, ASPIRIN WITH CODEINE #1, 2, 3, 4)

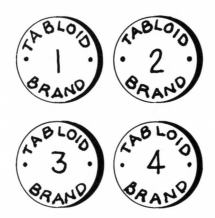

Codeine (Empirin)
No. 1 grl/8   No. 2 grl/4
No. 3 grl/2   No. 4 grl

Color: white

Purpose

Moderate pain relief.

Indications

For moderate pain relief over the short term.

Dosage

For some curious reason, the strengths of codeine are often coded in numbers. For example, Empirin with codeine #1 or just Empirin #1 contains one-eighth grain or 8 mg of codeine per tablet, #2 contains one-fourth grain or 16 mg, #3 contains one-half grain or 32 mg, and #4 contains one grain or 65 mg of codeine phosphate. A common dosage is a #3 tablet (32 mg codeine) every four hours as needed for pain.

Side Effects

The side effects are proportional to the dosage. The more you take, the more side effects you are likely to have. Allergic reactions are quite rare.

Codeine is a narcotic. Thus, it can lead to addiction, with tolerance and drug dependence. Frequently in persons with arthritis it leads to constipation and sometimes a set of complications including fecal impaction and diverticuli. More worrisome is the way that persons using codeine seem to lose their will to cope. The person taking codeine for many years sometimes seems sluggish and generally depressed. We don't really know if the codeine is responsible, but we do think that codeine often makes it more difficult for the person with arthritis to cope with the very real problems that abound.

PERCODAN (PERCOBARB, PERCOGESIC)

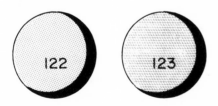

Percodan

Color: 0060-0122
light yellow

0060-0123 (Percodan-Demi)
pink

Purpose

For pain relief.

Indications

For short-term relief of moderate to severe pain.

Dosage

One tablet every six hours as needed.

Side Effects

Percodan is a curious combination drug. The basic narcotic is oxycodone, to which is added aspirin and other minor pain relievers. Combination drugs have a number of theoretical disadvantages, but Percodan is a strong and effective reliever of pain. It does require a special prescription because it is a strong narcotic and the hazards of serious addiction are present. The manufacturers state that that habit-forming potentialities are somewhat less than morphine and somewhat greater than codeine. The drug is usually well tolerated.

Special Hints

Percodan is a good drug for people with cancer, but it is very dangerous in the treatment of arthritis. It is not an anti-inflammatory agent and does not work directly on any of the disease processes. It is habit forming and it does break the pain reflex. It is a mental depressant and serious addiction can result.

DEMEROL (MEPERIDINE)

Purpose

For relief of severe pain.

Demerol

Color: pink/dark pink splotches

Indications

For temporary relief of severe pain, as with a bad fracture that has been immobilized.

Dosage

Various preparations come with 25 mg, 50 mg, or 100 mg of Demerol. One tablet every four hours for pain is a typical dose. Dose is increased for more severe pain and decreased for milder pain.

Side Effects

Demerol is a major narcotic approximately equivalent to morphine in pain relief and in addiction potential. Tolerance develops and increasing doses may be required. Drug dependence and severe withdrawal symptoms may be seen if the drug is stopped. Psychological dependence also occurs. The underlying disease may be covered up and serious symptoms may be masked. Nausea, vomiting, constipation, and a variety of other side effects may occur.

Special Hints

This is not a drug for the treatment of arthritis. Stay away from it.

TRANQUILIZERS

Valium, Librium, and other drugs of this ilk are the most-prescribed drugs in this country. They do not help arthritis, they act to depress the patient, and they should be avoided by persons with arthritis whenever possible.

AN EXTRA WORD ABOUT ASPIRIN AND MONEY

It is well known that aspirin is the best single drug for arthritis. However, there are many types of aspirin at many different prices and in combination with many different drugs. By knowing how to buy and reading labels, you can spend much less on your arthritis medications. In fact, the difference between the least expensive and the most expensive aspirin is nearly 67 dollars per year.

When buying, there are a few things to remember:

1. All you need is aspirin. The addition of such drugs as caffeine, which you find in Anacin, will do nothing for your arthritis.

2. Buffered aspirin or coated aspirin are always more expensive. Before buying, try all the hints for taking regular aspirin.

3. Tylenol or other drugs with acetaminophen *are not* the same as aspirin. They have *no effect* on the inflammation of joints.

The following prices were obtained at a well-known chain drugstore on Memorial Day 1980. While prices will change, the relative prices should remain about the same.

ASPIRIN AND ASPIRIN PRODUCTS

Drug Name	Number of Pills per Bottle	Content Each Pill	Price per 100	Price per Pill	Price of Equivalent of 8 5-gr Aspirin per Day for 1 Year
Anacin	100	Aspirin, 400 mg or 5.7 gr + 30 mg caffeine	2.09	.02	47.82
Anacin Arthritis Pain Formula	100	Aspirin, 7.5 gr or 486 mg + 2 antacids	3.83	.04	72.12
Anacin, Maximum Strength	100	Aspirin, 500 mg or 7.1 gr + 32 mg caffeine	2.89	.03	52.90
Bayer Aspirin	100	Asprin, 5 gr or 325 mg.	1.79	.02	50.41

Bayer Time Release Aspirin	125	Aspirin, 10 gr or 650 mg	3.67	.04	51.67
Bufferin	100	Aspirin, 5 gr or 324 mg + an antacid	2.09	.02	58.85
Bufferin, Arthritis Strength	100	Aspirin, 7.5 gr or 486 mg + an antacid	3.19	.03	60.07
Ecotrin	250	Aspirin, 5 gr or 325 mg	2.82	.03	79.41
Long's Aspirin	250	Aspirin, 5 gr or 325 mg	0.44	.003	12.39
Long's Buffered Aspirin	100	Aspirin, 5 gr or 325 mg + an antacid	1.09	.01	30.69
Norwich Aspirin	250	Aspirin, 5 gr or 325 mg	0.51	.005	14.08

NONASPIRIN PAIN RELIEVERS

Drug Name	Number of Pills per Bottle	Content Each Pill	Price per 100	Price per Pill	Price of Equivalent of 8 5-gr Aspirin per Day for 1 year
Anacin	30	500 mg acetaminophen + 32 mg caffeine	3.97	.04	72.67
Long's Acetaminophen	100	325 mg acetaminophen	1.39	.01	39.42
Tylenol	100	325 mg acetaminophen	2.09	.02	58.85
Tylenol Extra Strength	60	500 mg acetaminophen	4.82	.05	88.23

13
Working with Your Doctor
A JOINT VENTURE

CHOOSING A DOCTOR

There are many different kinds of doctors and sometimes it is difficult to know what kind to work with for what. Fortunately, most people with arthritis do not need a specialist. Therefore, it often is best to find a doctor who can help you with all of your health problems. For most of you, this will be an internist or a family practitioner.

An *internist* is a doctor who has had special training in the care of adults. Internists take care of all common adult health problems, including arthritis. A *family practitioner* has special training in taking care of all the common health problems that occur in a family. Thus a family practitioner may assist at the birth of a baby and also take care of grandmother's arthritis. As a general rule, the fewer doctors you have, the better coordinated your health care will be.

For people with difficult arthritis, a specialist might be the answer. If your arthritis is resistant to treatment or if you have severe rheumatoid arthritis, the expertise of a *rheumatologist* might be of value. Rheumatologists

173

are internists with additional training in arthritis and rheumatic diseases. To find a rheumatologist look in the yellow pages of your telephone book. (Unfortunately, not all communities have physicians listed by specialty.) You can also get a list of rheumatologists in your area from the nearest office of the Arthritis Foundation; these are listed immediately following this chapter. Finally, you can call your County Medical Society for a list of their members who are rheumatologists. Remember that not all doctors belong to the Medical Society.

Once you have a doctor, the next step is knowing if you are getting proper treatment. For instance, if your doctor says only, "You must expect some arthritis with aging" or "There is nothing that can be done" or "All that is wrong is a little arthritis," then you are probably not getting the best treatment and you may want to go to another doctor for a second opinion.

On the other hand, if your doctor suggests that you should take aspirin and exercise, you are probably getting good advice.

Also, don't get discouraged if your doctor has you experiment with several different treatment regimens. The proper combination of drugs, rest, and exercise is different for every person. Therefore, it may take a good deal of trial and error to find out what is best for you.

Finally, unless you have very serious symptoms, be cautious of taking prednisone. This is a very powerful drug with serious side effects and should not be used until most other drugs have been tried. It is almost never appropriate for osteoarthritis (see Chapter 12).

One last word about choosing a doctor. We have met persons who are upset because every doctor they see wants to start them on a different treatment. They want to know who is "right." The reality is that there is no right or wrong. Rather, each doctor has a little different approach as to where to start in the trial-and-error process of how to help you best. Therefore, select one doctor with whom you are comfortable and work with him or her. Only by forming a long-term relationship can you hope to get the best care. A problem with arthritis is usually long term and so must be your partnership with your doctor.

COMMUNICATING WITH YOUR DOCTOR

This is a huge area and probably causes more concern than anyone wishes to admit. Let us first examine expectations.

When someone goes to the doctor he or she usually wants relief of symptoms and/or reassurance that all is well. He or she may also want information about health or illness. On the other hand, the doctor wants the person to get well and usually feels that the best way to accomplish this is for him or her to follow the medical advice.

A shortened version of a typical encounter with a doctor might go something like this:

PATIENT: Doctor, I have a pain in my knee.

DOCTOR: How long have you had the pain? (Meanwhile, the knee is being examined.)

PATIENT: Six months.

DOCTOR: I think you have arthritis. I want you to exercise, take aspirin, and lose some weight. Let me know how you are feeling in a month or so.

PATIENT: Thank you doctor; I'll do that.

Meanwhile, the patient is thinking: "How much aspirin? Does he want me to jog at my age? What does weight have to do with all this? That is what he tells everyone. Why doesn't he give me some good medicine? He just wants to get rid of me."

And the doctor is thinking: "I know he or she won't do those things; my patients never do. I wish I knew how to get people to realize that aspirin, proper exercise, and weight control are the best treatment for osteoarthritis. Patients always want a miracle cure and we just don't have one."

The fact is that arthritis is a very frustrating disease for both doctor and patient because there is not any quick, easy answer.

Before continuing, let's look at some research about doctors and patients. Doctors think that patients ought to know a great deal about arthritis. They also believe that patients know very little. The reality is that patients know more than doctors think they know, but patients often don't ask questions or seek information.

Thus, there are three important things you can do to communicate with your doctor:

1. Ask questions. To be sure you don't forget, go to your appointment with a written list of questions. Don't wait for the doctor to ask for questions. Ask them when you first enter the office. Research has shown that it is important to ask questions early in the appointment. Later, if you don't understand something, ask. "How many aspirin?" "What kind of exercise?" "Why should I lose weight?" "What do you mean by *synovitis*?"

2. If for some reason you know you won't or can't follow the doctor's advice, let the doctor know. For example, "I won't take aspirin. It gives me stomach problems." "Clinoril may be good but I can't afford it." "I hate

exercise." "I would like to lose weight but I can't seem to give u
chocolate and need help."

Often, if your doctor knows why you can't or won't follow advic
alternate suggestions can be made to help you over the hump. If yo
don't share your problems there is no hope of finding solutions.

3. If you have problems with your treatment let your doctor know. Don't ju
   stop or change doctors. Since much arthritis treatment is trial and err
   you must work with your doctor.

If your doctor will not answer your questions or discuss your problem
you may want to think about finding another doctor. On the other hand, if yo
don't ask questions or communicate your problems, don't expect your doct
to read your mind. Contrary to popular opinion, a doctor is not God.

Finally, don't be afraid to ask financial questions. You have a right t
know how much an appointment will cost. You can ask the receptionist whe
you call the doctor's office. If you feel a treatment is too expensive, ask
there are any alternatives. For example, an exercise class at the YMCA c
senior citizen center may be as effective as working with a physical ther
pist. You may be able to test your own urine at home. There are almos
always solutions to such problems if they are discussed.

In short, to get the most from your doctor, be a CAD:

Come prepared, **A**sk questions, **D**iscuss problems

A doctor's addendum: I never have seen a person with arthritis that
couldn't help. There are some individuals, however, that I have not helpec
In every such case, the communication broke down. Sometimes I am short c
time or short of temper. Sometimes the person doesn't listen or doesn't hea
or doesn't understand. Often, a preconceived opinion is the problem. "Aspiri
won't work." "My neighbor couldn't tolerate that drug." "I hardly eat
thing." "She seems too old to exercise." "I don't think he would understand.
Or a person who reports being worse never filled a prescription, stopped a
exercise program after two days, decreased medication ("It was too exper
sive"), and never mentioned the problem. A solid half of the blame lies wit
the doctor. Sometimes we do not listen or have our own preconceived idea
No matter how hard we try we don't always get it right. But the other half c
the blame lies with the patient. Tell it true and straight and we can help. Thi
is a partnership. We don't always have to agree to get good results. But th
give-and-take of direct communication is essential.

THE ARTHRITIS FOUNDATION

The "AF" is a truly marvelous institution. It sponsors programs in public education and professional education, supports young doctors establishing research careers in arthritis, and provides direct support for research activities. The meetings of the American Rheumatism Association (ARA), a section of the Arthritis Foundation, provide the principle forum for discussion of new scientific knowledge about arthritis. The AF leads the fight for increased government programs of research and service.

The Arthritis Foundation consists of a national office and local chapters around the country. You will usually want to contact the local chapter, which can advise you of doctors and clinics in your area, provide instructional materials, and occasionally may be able to help with financial problems. There may be a schedule of activities you might wish to attend. Or you might want to volunteer your efforts in support of the chapter.

National Office
The Arthritis Foundation
1314 Spring St., N.W.
Atlanta, Georgia 30309
Telephone: (404) 266-0795

ARTHRITIS FOUNDATION CHAPTERS

Alabama

Alabama Chapter
13 Office Park Circle—Room 14
Birmingham, Alabama 35223
205-870-4700

South Alabama Chapter
304 Little Flower Avenue
Mobile, Alabama 36606
205-471-1725

Arizona

Central Arizona Chapter
2102 West Indian School Road—Suite 9
Phoenix, Arizona 85015
602-264-7679

Southern Arizona Chapter
3813 East Second Street
Tucson, Arizona 85716
602-326-2811

Arkansas

Arkansas Chapter
6213 Lee Avenue
Little Rock, Arkansas 72205
501-664-7242

California

Northeastern California Chapter
1722 "J" Street—Suite 321
Sacramento, California 95814
916-446-7246

Northern California Chapter
185 Berry Street—Building 3, Suite 363
San Francisco, California 94107
415-974-1566

San Diego Area Chapter
6154 Mission Gorge Road—Suite 110
San Diego, California 92120
714-280-0304

Southern California Chapter
4311 Wilshire Boulevard
Los Angeles, California 90010
213-938-6111

Colorado

Rocky Mountain Chapter
234 Columbine Street—Suite 210
Denver, Colorado 80206
303-399-5065

Connecticut

Connecticut Chapter
929 Silas Deane Highway
Wethersfield, Connecticut 06109
203-563-1177

Delaware

Delaware Chapter
234 Philadelphia Pike—Suite 1
Wilmington, Delaware 19809
302-764-8254

District of Columbia

Metropolitan Washington Chapter
2424 Pennsylvania Ave. N.W. #105
Washington, D.C. 20037
202-331-7395

Florida

Florida Chapter
3205 Manatee Ave. West
Bradenton, Florida 33505
813-748-1300

Georgia

Georgia Chapter
2799 Delk Road, S.E.
Marietta, Georgia 30067
404-952-4254

Metropolitan Branch
C&S Northeast Center
2059 Coolridge Road

Tucker, Georgia 30084
404-491-1558

Hawaii
Hawaii Chapter
200 North Vineyard—Suite 505
Honolulu, Hawaii 96817
808-531-1920

Idaho
Idaho Chapter
700 Robbins Road—Suite 1
Boise, Idaho 83702
208-344-7102

Illinois
Central Illinois Chapter
Allied Agencies Center
320 East Armstrong Ave.—Rm. 102
Peoria, Illinois 61603
309-672-6337

Illinois Chapter
79 W. Monroe—Suite 1105
Chicago, Illinois 60603
312-782-1367

Indiana
Indiana Chapter
1010 East 86th Street
Indianapolis, Indiana 46240
317-844-3341

Iowa
Iowa Chapter
1501 Ingersoll Ave.—Suite 101
Des Moines, Iowa 50309
515-243-6259

Kansas
Kansas Chapter
1602 East Waterman
Wichita, Kansas 67211
316-263-0116

Kentucky
Kentucky Chapter
1381 Bardstown Road
Louisville, Kentucky 40204
502-459-6460

Louisiana
Louisiana Chapter
4700 Dryades
New Orleans, Louisiana 70115
504-897-1338

Maine
Maine Chapter
37 Mill Street
Brunswick, Maine 04011
207-729-4453

Maryland
Maryland Chapter
12 West 25th Street
Baltimore, Maryland 21218
301-366-0923

Massachusetts
Massachusetts Chapter
59 Temple Place
Boston, Massachusetts 02111
617-542-6535

Michigan
Michigan Chapter
23400 Michigan Ave.—Suite 605
Dearborn, Michigan 48124
313-561-9096

Minnesota
Minnesota Chapter
122 West Franklin—Suite 440
Minneapolis, Minnesota 55404
612-874-1201

Mississippi
Mississippi Chapter
6055 Ridgewood Road
Jackson, Mississippi 39211
601-956-3371

Missouri
Eastern Missouri Chapter
4144 Lindell Boulevard
St. Louis, Missouri 63108
314-533-1324

Greater Kansas City Chapter
8301 State Line Road—Suite 117
Kansas City, Missouri 64114
913-361-7002

Montana
Montana Chapter
P.O. Box 20994
Billings, Montana 59104
406-652-1538

Nebraska
Nebraska Chapter
120 North 69th Street—Room 202
Omaha, Nebraska 68132
402-558-2400

Nevada
Nevada Division
2700 State Street—14A
Las Vegas, Nevada 89104
702-369-8102

New Hampshire
New Hampshire Chapter
P.O. Box 369
Concord, New Hampshire 03301
603-224-9322

New Jersey
New Jersey Chapter
15 Prospect Street

Colonia, New Jersey 07067
201-388-0744

New Mexico
New Mexico Chapter
5112 Grand Avenue, N.E.
Albuquerque, New Mexico 87108
505-265-1545

New York
Central New York Chapter
505 East Fayette Street—Second floor
Syracuse, New York 13212
315-422-8174

Genesee Valley Chapter
973 East Avenue
Rochester, New York 14607
716-271-3540

Long Island Division
501 Walt Whitman Road
Melville, New York 11747
516-427-8272

New York Chapter
221 Park Avenue South
New York, New York 10003
212-677-5790

Northeastern New York Chapter
1237 Central Avenue
Albany, New York 12205
518-459-5082

Western New York Chapter
4556 Bailey Avenue
Buffalo, New York 14226
716-837-8600

North Carolina
North Carolina Chapter
P.O. Box 2505
Durham, North Carolina 27705
919-477-0286

North Dakota

Dakota Chapter
402 N. 39th St.
Fargo, North Dakota 58102
701-282-3653

Ohio

Akron Area Chapter
26 Locust Street
Akron, Ohio 44302
216-253-1171

Central Ohio Chapter
501 N. Star Road
Columbus, Ohio 43221
614-488-0777

Northeastern Ohio Chapter
11416 Bellflower Road
Cleveland, Ohio 44106
216-791-1310

Northwestern Ohio Chapter
447 Talmadge Road
Toledo, Ohio 43623
419-473-3349

Southwestern Ohio Chapter
7400 Reading Road
Cincinnati, Ohio 45202
513-721-1027

Oklahoma

Eastern Oklahoma Chapter
4615-D South Memorial
Tulsa, Oklahoma 74129
918-622-0639

Oklahoma Chapter
3313 Classen Boulevard—Suite 101
Oklahoma City, Oklahoma 73118
405-521-0066

Oregon

Oregon Chapter
3330 N.W. Flanders—Suite 207

Portland, Oregon 92207
503-222-7246

Pennsylvania

Central Pennsylvania Chapter
P.O. Box 668
Camp Hill, Pennsylvania 17011
717-763-0900

Eastern Pennsylvania Chapter
311 So. Juniper Street—Suite 201
Philadelphia, Pennsylvania 19107
215-735-5272

Western Pennsylvania Chapter
2201 Clark Building
Pittsburgh, Pennsylvania 15222
412-566-1645

Rhode Island

Rhode Island Chapter
850 Waterman Avenue
East Providence, Rhode Island 02914
401-434-5792

South Carolina

South Carolina Chapter
3008 Millwood Avenue
Columbia, South Carolina 29205
803-254-6702

South Dakota (see **North Dakota**)

Tennessee

Middle-East Tennessee Chapter
1719 West End Building
Nashville, Tennessee 37203
615-329-3431

West Tennessee Chapter
2600 Poplar Avenue—Suite 200
Memphis, Tennessee 38112
901-452-4482

Texas

North Texas Chapter
5415 Maple Avenue—Suite 417
Dallas, Texas 75235
214-638-7474

Northwest Texas Chapter
3145 McCart Avenue
Fort Worth, Texas 76110
817-926-7733

South Central Texas Chapter
503 S. Main Street
San Antonio, Texas 78204
512-224-4857

Texas Gulf Coast Chapter
9099-A Katy Freeway
Houston, Texas 77024
713-468-6572

West Texas Chapter
1926 34th Street
Lubbock, Texas 79401
806-747-5125

Utah

Utah Chapter
Graystone Plaza, #4
1174 E. 2700 South
Salt Lake City, Utah 84106
801-486-4993

Vermont

Vermont Chapter
215 College Street

Burlington, Vermont 05401
802-864-4988

Virginia

Peninsula Branch
12388 Warwick Boulevard—Suite 102
Newport News, Virginia 23606
804-872-8848

Virginia Chapter
P.O. Box 6772
Richmond, Virginia 23230
804-282-5491

Washington

Western Washington Chapter
726 Broadway—Suite 103
Seattle, Washington 98122
206-324-9940

West Virginia

West Virginia Chapter
P.O. Box 8473
South Charleston, W. Va. 25303
304-744-3042

Wisconsin

Wisconsin Chapter
1442 N. Farwell Avenue—Suite 508
Milwaukee, Wisconsin 53202
414-276-0490
Toll-free 1-800-242-9945

Wyoming (see **Colorado**)

BIBLIOGRAPHY

nson, Herbert. **The Relaxation Response.** New York: Avon Books, 1976.

ggs, Jo-An. **Living and Loving with Arthritis—Information on Sex and hritis.** Arthritis Center of Hawaii, 347 No. Kuakini Street, Honolulu, waii 96817.

mfort, Alex. **The Joy of Sex.** New York: Simon and Schuster, 1972.

wning, George. **The Massage Book.** New York: Random House, 1972.

es, James F., M.D. **Arthritis. A Comprehensive Guide.** Reading, Mass.: dison-Wesley, 1979.

ce, Gay Gaer, and Julius Segal. **Troubled Sleep.** Garden City, N.Y.: ubleday, 1969.

ntell, Robert H., M.D., James F. Fries, M.D., and Donald M. Vickery, M.D. **king Care of Your Child.** Reading, Mass.: Addison-Wesley, 1977.

rbo, Richard. **How to Get a Good Night's Sleep.** Boston: Little, Brown, 1978.

kery, Donald M., M.D., and James F. Fries, M.D. **Take Care of Yourself.** ading, Mass.: Addison-Wesley, 1976.

Watson, David, and Roland Thorp. **Self-Directed Behavior: Self-Modificat** **for Personal Adjustment.** 2d ed. Monterey, Calif.: Brooks/Cole, 1977.

White, John, and James Fadiman, eds. **Relax.** New York: Confucian Pr◄ 1976.

NUTRITION

General Nutrition

McGill, Marion, and Orrea Pye. **The No-Nonsense Guide to Food and Nutriti◄** New York: Butterick, 1978.

Vegetarian Eating

Lappe, Frances M. **Diet for a Small Planet.** New York: Ballantine, 1976.

Robertson, Laurel, Carol Flinders, and Bronween Godfrey. **Laurel's Kitch◄** New York: Milgiri/Bantam, 1976.

Weight Control

Ferguson, James M. **Habits, Not Diets.** Palo Alto, Calif.: Bull, 1976.

Stuart, Richard B., and Barbara Davis. **Slim Chance in a Fat World.** Cha◄ paign, Ill.: Research Press, 1972.

INDEX